YOUTH WITH IMPULSE-CONTROL
DISORDERS

On the Spur of
the Moment

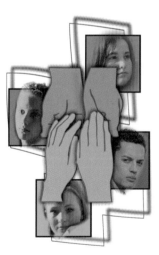

HELPING YOUTH WITH MENTAL, PHYSICAL, AND SOCIAL CHALLENGES

Title List

YOUTH WITH IMPULSE-CONTROL
DISORDERS

On the Spur of
the Moment

by Kenneth McIntosh
and Phyllis Livingston

Mason Crest Publishers
Philadelphia

Mason Crest Publishers Inc.
370 Reed Road
Broomall, Pennsylvania 19008
(866) MCP-BOOK (toll free)
www.masoncrest.com

First printing

1 2 3 4 5 6 7 8 9 10

ISBN 978-1-4222-0133-6 (series)

Library of Congress Cataloging-in-Publication Data

McIntosh, Kenneth.
  Youth with impulse-control disorders : on the spur of the moment / by Kenneth McIntosh and Phyllis Livingston.
      p. cm. — (Helping youth with mental, physical, and social challenges)
  Includes bibliographical references and index.
    ISBN 978-1-4222-0147-3 (alk. paper)
    1. Impulse control disorders in children—Juvenile literature. I. Livingston, Phyllis, 1957– II. Title.
RJ506.I5M375 2008
618.92'8584—dc22
2006038604

Interior pages produced by
Harding House Publishing Service, Inc.
www.hardinghousepages.com
Interior design by MK Bassett-Harvey.
Cover design by MK Bassett-Harvey.
Cover Illustration by Keith Rosko.
Printed in the Hashemite Kingdom of Jordan.

The creators of this book have made every effort to provide accurate information, but it should not be used as a substitute for the help and services of trained professionals.

Contents

Introduction

We are all people first, before anything else. Our shared humanity is more important than the impressions we give to each other by how we look, how we learn, or how we act. Each of us is worthy simply because we are all part of the human race. Though we are all different in many ways, we can celebrate our differences as well as our similarities.

In this book series, you will read about many young people with various special needs that impact their lives in different ways. The disabilities are not *who* the people are, but the disabilities are an important characteristic of each person. When we recognize that we all have differing needs, we can grow toward greater awareness and tolerance of each other. Just as important, we can learn to accept our differences.

Not all young people with a disability are the same as the persons in the stories. But you will learn from these stories how a special need impacts a young person, as well as his or her family and friends. The story will help you understand differences better and appreciate how differences make us all stronger and better.

—*Cindy Croft, M.A.Ed.*

6

Did you know that as many as 8 percent of teens experience anxiety or depression, and as many as 70 to 90 percent will use substances such as alcohol or illicit drugs at some time? Other young people are living with life-threatening diseases including HIV infection and cancer, as well as chronic psychiatric conditions such as bipolar disease and schizophrenia. Still other teens have the challenge of being "different" from peers because they are intellectually gifted, are from another culture, or have trouble controlling their behavior or socializing with others. All youth with challenges experience additional stresses compared to their typical peers. The good news is that there are many resources and supports available to help these young people, as well as their friends and families.

The stories contained in each book of this series also contain factual information that will enhance your own understanding of the particular condition being presented. If you or someone you know is struggling with a similar condition or experience, this series can give you important information about where and how you can get help. After reading these stories, we hope that you will be more open to the differences you encounter in your peers and more willing to get to know others who are "different."

—*Carolyn Bridgemohan, M.D.*

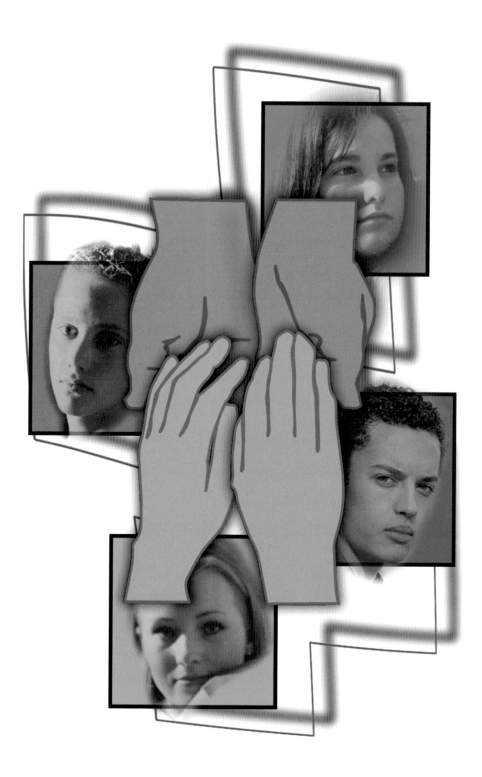

Chapter 1

Girl with a Secret

She's the girl everyone at Shore View High envies. But she has a shameful secret no one else knows.

Vanna Khan drives her pink Acura into the school parking lot; it's a good half hour before classes start, so she'll have plenty of time to socialize. She looks in the mirror: every hair is in place, and the bright California morning sun gleams off the blond highlights in her hair. *Lip gloss? Check. Eyeliner? Check. Perfect.*

She turns to her little sister in the passenger seat. "Need a ride home today, M'liss?"

"I'm set, Vann. I'll get a ride home with Carlos."

"Okay, but watch yourself. Those Mexican boys just want one thing. And you're only a freshman."

M'liss sticks her tongue out. "Has it ever occurred to you that Mexicans probably stay stuff like that about us Cambodians?"

"Maybe, but you should listen to your big sister."

"Yeah. Right, my big sister who flirts with every boy at Shore View High."

"I flirt—but that's as far as it goes. They can look but not touch. I'm popular, our family keeps their honor, and everything's cool." Vanna flashes a smug smile. "Now, get out of the car. I've gotta park and get in there to see people."

M'liss jumps out, grabs her backpack, and heads for the door. Vanna notices her sister is wearing a brown Roxy top with black jeans. *Bad color choice*, Vanna tells herself. *I've gotta give M'liss more fashion advice.*

She parks the Acura and steps out. Her own clothes are chosen more carefully: form-fitting yellow pants from the Fashion Boutique in Laguna and a white blouse custom tailored to fit her surgically enhanced breasts. From the tips of her manicured fingernails to the bottom of her high heels, Vanna looks good and she knows it.

She heads toward the school entrance, hips swaying slightly, head straight upright. As Vanna greets her fellow students, she makes a mental note of their status within the school.

"Hello, Josh."

"Hey, Vanna."

Josh Bruner—some girls call him Boy Wonder, but he's not that great. Nice ripped bod, and he's popular, attractive in a caveman sort of way. He's going steady with Ashley Gordon, who is mousey, and what does a boy so good looking see in her? But, there's no accounting for taste and he's a surfer boy, and Ashley's a surfer girl, so it kinda makes sense.

Vanna recalls her few experiences playing in the ocean. *Boogie board flipped over and I swallowed this horrible tasting saltwater. It ruined my hair for days afterward, and I got surf wax and sand all over a hundred-dollar bikini. Water sports are so not for me.*

"Hiya, Vanna."

"Hey, Jason."

Jason Hughes, lead guitarist and singer for the local band Impulse. He's so cute, we could be a thing. But he's a pot head— bad for my reputation. So give him winks, keep him interested, and someday, who knows? She winks at him, and Jason stares after her like a starved man eyeing a triple hamburger. He's so absorbed that he walks right into an oncoming student.

"Hey! Watch it!"

"Whoa, sorry dude."

Thinking about Jason, smiling a little, Vanna absent-mindedly brushes against Kyle Brown. He's a geek: lives on his computer and Playstation. He doesn't even register on the social scale, so Vanna doesn't waste mental energy thinking about him.

She struts through the school entrance and heads for the stairs in the main hallway. The people who matter are already there.

"Hey, Vann."

"Hey yourself, Stacie."

Stacie Combs, part of the inner circle. Bleached blond and thin as a rail, her parents are both doctors. She's annoying sometimes, but about as good a friend as one could hope for in this town.

"What's up, Vanna?"

"Just arriving, Jaynee."

Jaynee Mendez, she's uber-hip, the only real competition here when it comes to fashion. She's actually gained some weight lately, but all the boys still think she's hot, so go figure. Gotta hang with her to be popular.

The three girls are just catching up on the day's gossip when they are unexpectedly interrupted.

KABOOM! There's a sudden loud bang and the sound of shattered glass, followed by panicked screams.

The three girls turn toward the sound and see students running their way.

"Hey! What happened?" yells Stacie.

An underclassman stops and gives a rapid reply. "Fire in the chem lab! The window just blew out, and there are flames in the hallway."

His words are cut short by the shriek of the school fire alarm. Students run pell-mell for the exits. Vanna, Stacie, and Jaynee walk calmly toward the door. *Just because it's an emergency doesn't mean we should lose our composure. Panicked people are not cool.*

There's a buzz of voices outside the school on the front lawn. The girls join the others, all three looking bored.

Kyle Brown walks up to the trio. "Hey, Vanna, Stacie, Jaynee—what do you think caused that?"

It's not good to be talking to Kyle Brown—he is totally not with it. But it's rude not to answer someone standing right in front of you.

"I dunno, Kyle. What do you think?"

"Well, I think someone must've started a fire. Things don't just ignite by themselves."

Why do eggheads like Kyle say things so stupidly obvious?

"Yeah, that makes sense. See ya, Kyle." *Will he get the clue that this conversation is over?*

"See ya, girls." He walks away.

Fire trucks are arriving, and a few minutes later the school principal stands on the steps to the front entrance to make an announcement. Her voice sounds tinny through the bullhorn. "Students, school is closed for the day. You are dismissed. Come back at the normal time tomorrow."

Police cars are pulling up. *Kyle's right: they're closing school so they can do some kind of investigation.*

"Hey, Vanna, wanna drive up to Rodeo Drive and spend the morning shopping?" Jaynee asks.

"Yeah, that's cool."

Vanna and Jaynee climb into Jaynee's black Jeep Cherokee and join the line heading out of the parking lot. Vanna sees M'liss heading toward a car holding hands with Carlos Figueroa. *Watch yourself M'liss: it would be awful if people thought my little sister was acting like a slut. Do what makes you happy, but don't get caught.* Vanna waves and the pair wave back at her.

SCREECH! Jaynee hits the brakes just in time to prevent hitting a girl stepping in front of the Jeep. The girl grimaces, mouthing the word, "Sorry!"

"Hey, watch it!" Jaynee yells out the window.

"Don't be too hard on her, Jaynee" Vanna says. "That's the new girl, Tanya Begay. She's a Navajo Indian. She used to live on a reservation in Arizona."

"She should watch where she's going, though."

She's not used to So Cal. Everything is different where she comes from. Vanna's mind replays images from when she was in first grade, with out-of-style clothes and pigtails, and some of the kids called her "Gook." Ten years later, it still gives her chills remembering that. She also pictures her parents. They live in a great deco-style house near the beach, so Vanna doesn't have to be embarrassed telling friends where she lives. But she is still uncomfortable when her parents try to talk with her friends; they have strong accents and keep talking about "back in Cambodia" or quoting Buddhist sages. *So not cool.*

Vanna tells herself, *Kids should give this Begay girl a break. Give her a year or two and she'll get with the scene. I did it; she will too. She'll be the queen of Shore View High and no one will make fun of her.*

Two hours later the girls are shopping in All That Glitters, a trendy fashion store on Rodeo Drive. Jaynee is in the dressing room, trying on a pair of pants. Vanna spies a pink tube top on the sales rack. *That would look cute on me,* she thinks.

All of a sudden she's uncomfortable, sweaty. Her hands are trembling. Vanna looks carefully around the store. *Is there a surveillance cam? There it is. It faces away from this rack, so it won't see me. Any store guards? Nope. Just one other customer, and no way that old lady is security. Is the cashier looking? She's on the phone with her back toward me. Good.*

With a practiced, liquid motion, Vanna reaches out to the rack, twirls the tube top around her right hand, and slips the hand into her big purse. She smoothly deposits the item of clothing in the bottom of her handbag. It only takes a moment; you would hardly see these motions if you were looking straight at her.

Vanna feels more relaxed now, like a person who has just gotten over the urge to make an embarrassing sneeze. She wonders, *Why do I keep doing this? It's not like I can't afford the clothes I want—and I don't even want these things that badly. Half the stuff I steal I give away; sometimes I just drop stuff in the trash and don't even wear it. If I ever got caught it would be so embarrassing. . . . But I don't get caught, not ever. And it feels so good afterward.*

This is Vanna's little secret.

It won't be a secret much longer, though.

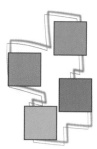

What Is an Impulse?

An impulse is an urge or desire that comes on suddenly without prior consideration. People feel both emotional and physical impulses. For example, if you're having a great time with your best friend, you might feel a sudden impulse to give her a hug. When watching your favorite soccer team score a goal, you might jump up and cheer. If you see somebody else get sick, you might feel unexpectedly nauseated yourself. Waking up from a bad dream, you could feel an abrupt need to switch on a light. These are all examples of common emotional impulses.

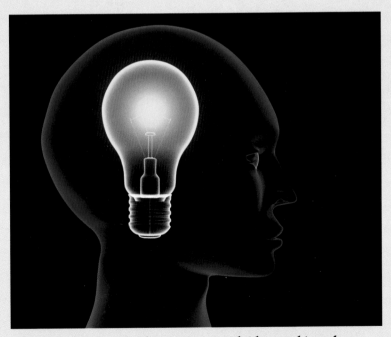

Our brains are constantly coming up with ideas and impulses—but in most cases, we do not feel compelled to act on each and every idea that occurs to us. A person with an impulse-control disorder, however, may experience these mental impulses as nearly irresistible.

In addition to these emotional impulses that you generally experience consciously, you are also experiencing unconscious physical impulses all the time. Your brain constantly sends messages causing you to breathe, blink, move your hands, walk, and perform all the other functions of your body. These impulses are necessary for your survival, but you don't have to think about them in order to make them happen.

However, many other impulses require that you make conscious responses. You feel the impulse to go to the bathroom, for instance, but then you must control the impulse until you are able to get to a restroom. You could get angry with your teacher and feel an impulse to yell at him, but you stop yourself because you know that yelling will get you into trouble. Sometimes you may find it easier to control an impulse than at other times. Every once in a while, you may even lose control of an impulse that you know you should have resisted. This happens to everyone to a certain degree and is a normal part of life. Some people, however, lose so much control over certain impulses that they develop an impulse-control disorder. Losing control over a single impulse, however, even a very serious one, does not automatically mean that you have an impulse-control disorder.

When people have impulse-control disorders, many of the impulses they might normally be able to control become so strong that they may seem irresistible. Often, this is because of neurological or chemical abnormalities in the brain; for these people,

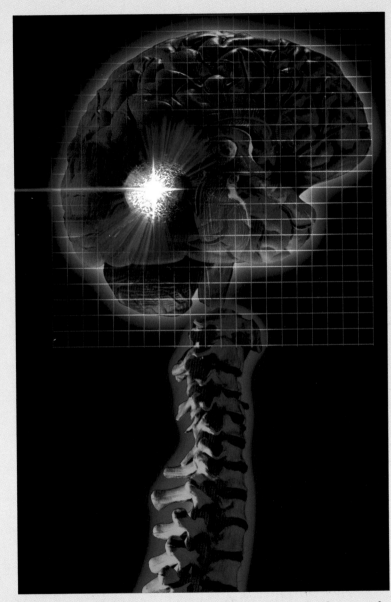

Brain function plays an important role in behavior. In the case of impulse-control disorders, the brain sends out insistent, repetitive messages.

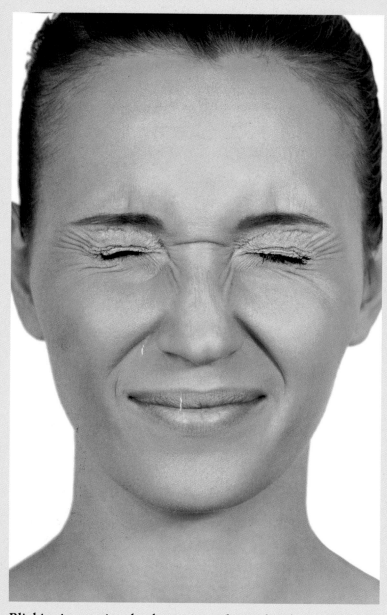

Blinking is an action that happens involuntarily—but one that most of us can also choose to control consciously. A person with a tic, however, might be compelled to blink over and over.

their urges truly are irresistible, and these urges happen to them frequently, not just occasionally. In the book *Handbook of Childhood Impulse Disorders and ADHD: Theory and Practice,* Leonard F. Koziol uses the example of a "tic" to explain what these types of impulses are like. A tic is an involuntary movement in a part of the body that a person would normally be able to control. For example, one's eyelid may spasm uncontrollably, or the muscles at the corner of a person's mouth may periodically contract, pulling the person's lips into a grimace. Koziol explains that the behavioral impulses associated with impulse-control disorders can be thought of as the result of a mental tic. The brain sends out repetitive, tic-like commands to perform certain actions. The person can lose so much conscious control over the impulsive action that she may not even realize what she is doing until after she has done it.

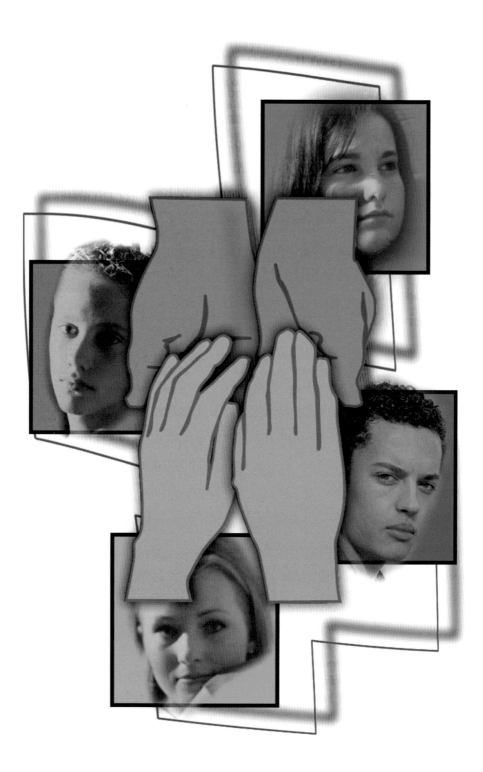

Chapter 2

Caught in the Act

Saturday afternoon Vanna is shopping again, this time at Seal Beach with Stacie. Tourists and locals crowd the sidewalks, and cars jostle for parking spots along the main street. Two sets of circumstances that work well for shoplifters: when stores are totally empty so no one is looking, and when stores are full of customers, so one can get away with theft due to the confusion of the crowds.

"Hey, Vanna," Stacie says, "I need a new sweatshirt. I'm gonna stop in at Harbor Style Surf Shop and see what they have."

"Okay. I'll be at Bikini Boutique."

Vanna enters the shop and looks through the racks. Her eyes fall on a shimmering blue swimsuit. She holds her arm next to it: *Nice contrast with my skin tone.* She holds up the top. *Eye-catching but not skanky; it's hard to find suits like that.*

Vanna notices her hand is shaking slightly, and she feels her heart pounding harder. *There's the feeling again.* She looks around the store; there are at least a dozen customers, all occupied with their own pursuits. The lady who works in the store is frantically dashing about trying to help all the customers.

Vanna takes the swimsuit and heads into the dressing room, slides off her sweatshirt and jeans, and tries on the suit. *Very nice. Hmm . . . I really need to look into modeling as a career.*

Vanna leaves the swimsuit on and pulls her clothes over it. She looks again in the mirror. *Good, no one can tell. As far as everyone in this store is concerned, I'm walking out without any items. Ahh . . . I'm feeling much better now.*

Vanna slides out of the dressing room and strides calmly out the front door of the shop onto the sidewalk.

"Vanna Khan, what are you doing?!" Vanna spins around, surprised by the voice behind her. It's Ashley Gordon, a brunette girl about her own size. *Josh Bruner's girlfriend: surfer crowd, not very good-looking, poor thing.*

Vanna assumes her sugary sweet voice. "Oh, hello, Ashley. How are you, hon?"

"Don't hon me. I saw what you did."

"Why Ashley, what on earth are you talking about?"

"You just stole a swimsuit."

Vanna's jaw drops. "How dare you?!"

"You took a swimsuit into the dressing room. I was waiting for the room and went in after you—there was no suit in the room and no suit in your hand. So you must be wearing it."

Vanna grows suddenly furious. "Who do you think you are, the store cop?"

Ashley shakes her head. "What kind of example are you setting for your little sister?"

"Don't lecture me," Vanna snaps back.

Ashley's voice grows quieter. "Your parents are rich, Vanna. You get everything you want. Why do you need to steal stuff?"

Vanna is so startled by Ashley's words that she finds herself answering truthfully. "I don't know why I steal, Ashley. I don't understand it. For real. I get all sweaty and nervous and . . . well, I feel better afterward."

Ashley's forehead wrinkles. "You don't have any idea why you do it?"

Vanna shakes her head and stares at the ground nervously. "Ashley, would you like a blue bikini?" *That was stupid. But I don't know what else to say.*

Ashley cracks a smile. "C'mon, Vanna. If the top fits you, it's twice too big for me. And no, I don't want stolen anything. And in case you're wondering, no—I am not getting back at you, although you have been pretty rough on me in the past."

"Sorry." Vanna is still staring at the ground, unable to lift her gaze to Ashley's face. "I'm a witch."

"Yeah, you can be rude sometimes. But that's not why I'm talking to you."

Vanna glances up from the sidewalk at last and looks into Ashley's eyes. She's surprised to find that they are filled with compassion.

"Vanna, you know how bad I was feeling six months ago. Depression was killing me, literally. I hated my life, everything about it."

A feeling of regret comes over Vanna, like a horrible monster crawling out of its lair. She feels tears swelling in the corners of her eyes. "Ashley, I treated you like crap when you were really hurting. I—I'm sorry."

Ashley shrugs. "Vanna, that doesn't matter. I'm not telling you this to make you feel bad. I'm trying to do you a favor."

Vanna stands frozen like a statue. *Since when does anyone from school do me a favor?*

Ashley continues, "When I had those problems I thought it was all my fault, that I was weird and no one would understand me. But I was wrong. Josh put me in contact with

Dr. Graham; she's a psychologist with the Redondo Medical Group. Dr. Graham is really cool, and she helped me get my life back together. I'm just thinking, maybe she could help you, too."

Vanna feels something click inside of her, confidence returning—the hideous monster called shame is slinking back into its lair defeated. She takes a breath, straightens her back, and glares at Ashley. Her bravado restored, she practically shouts at the other girl, "You want *me* to see a shrink?"

"Just making a suggestion."

"Shrinks are for people with problems. I don't have any problems."

Ashley frowns. "But you just said . . . ."

"What a joke! I don't need a freaking head doctor. Those are for people who are all messed up—like you!"

Vanna swirls around and strides into Harbor Style Surf Shop. Stacie is looking at a sweatshirt covered with hibiscus patterns. "Hey, Vanna, find anything at Bikini Boutique?"

"Nah, nothing."

Vanna glances out the window and watches Ashley walk away down the street.

That was crazy. I don't think she'll tell anyone, but who knows?

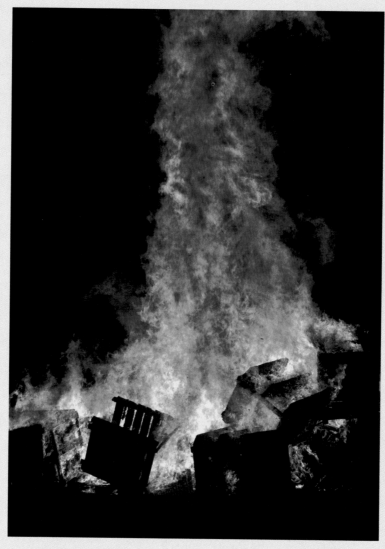

An individual with pyromania feels irresistible urges to start fires. Most people with this rare disorder are males who have an imbalance in their brain chemistry. Researchers have also linked pyromania to a history of child abuse. People with pyromania typically feel loneliness and isolation, which builds into a rage that is released and changed into euphoria when they start a fire.

Types of Impulse-Control Disorders

There are a number of different types of impulse-control disorders. Each one has a specific set of **criteria** to help doctors determine if the patient has an impulse-control disorder or if his behavior is caused by some other circumstance in his life.

Many psychiatric disorders involve a loss of impulse control. Eating disorders, obsessive-compulsive disorder, attention-deficit/hyperactivity disorder, and substance abuse are all characterized by an inability to control certain impulses. However, each of these has its own category and designation in the *Diagnostic and Statistical Manual of Mental Disorders*, Fourth Edition (called the DSM-IV).

The medical field recognizes five specific impulse-control disorders that exist independently of these other categories. They are:

1. **intermittent** explosive disorder

2. kleptomania

3. pyromania

4. **pathological** gambling

5. trichotillomania

Some people experience **chronic** difficulties in controlling impulses that are not part of these five specific disorders or any other category of mental disorder, but that are still serious enough to be considered disorders. For these people, there is another category called impulse-control disorder not otherwise specified.

Intermittent Explosive Disorder

A person with intermittent explosive disorder often has aggressive impulses that he cannot resist and that cause him to destroy property or hurt others. Many people overreact when they are angry, but they do not have intermittent explosive disorder. Lots of people may express extreme anger by slamming a fist on a table or yelling—but a person with intermittent explosive disorder acts out far more violently, destroying objects of value and threatening to harm or actually harming others. Furthermore, the person's actions are completely out of proportion with the situation. For example, someone might be justifiably angry to find that her car has a flat tire and might even kick the vehicle. The person with intermittent explosive disorder, however, would experience anger that is inappropriate for the situation. Perhaps she would begin screaming at other people in the car, putting dents in the vehicle, and threatening to drive the car over a cliff.

Many things can cause someone to overreact when she is angry. For example, people with psychiatric conditions like **borderline personality disorder** or **bipolar disorder** may have inappropriate reactions to certain situations. In order to be diagnosed with intermittent explosive disorder, the person's actions must not be caused by any other disorders, substance abuse, or **extenuating** circumstances.

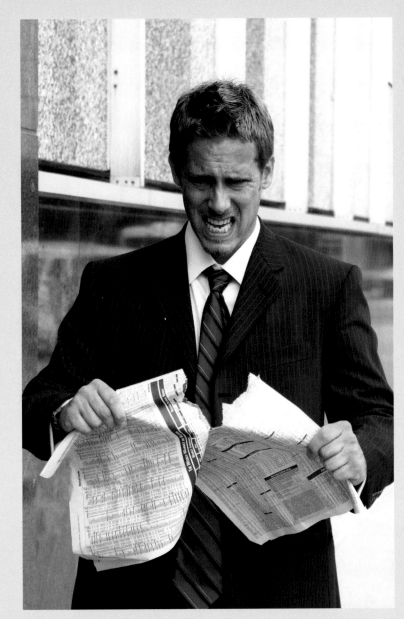

A person with intermittent explosive disorder often overreacts to life's everyday frustrations.

While aggressive and violent acts are increasingly common in our society, medically diagnosable intermittent explosive disorder seems to be rare. It occurs in men more often than in women. There is a lack of reliable research into the causes, onset, and course of intermittent explosive disorder, but the information that is available suggests that people develop the disorder between childhood and their early twenties. Furthermore, different people experience the disorder in very different ways. When it comes to treatment, some people respond very well to psychiatric therapy; other people find medication helpful; and still others receive very little relief from either of these forms of intervention.

Kleptomania

Kleptomania is an impulse-control disorder in which a person repeatedly steals. If a person repeatedly steals things he needs or wants but cannot afford, however, he does not have kleptomania. People with kleptomania steal things they do not need and that usually have very little monetary value. They often throw away the objects or give them away as gifts soon after stealing them. The person with kleptomania feels a growing sense of tension or internal chaos before stealing. Directly after stealing, he feels a sense of relief, as though the tension has broken. In order for a diagnosis of kleptomania to be made, a doctor must determine that the stealing is not caused by another condition (like **hallucinations** or a personality disorder), is not done to express anger or vengeance, and is not caused by the influence of drugs or alcohol.

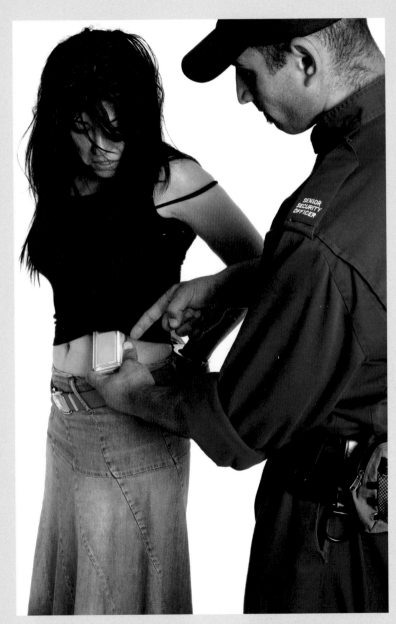

A person who steals objects she doesn't really need, simply because it helps her to release tension and feel better emotionally, may have kleptomania.

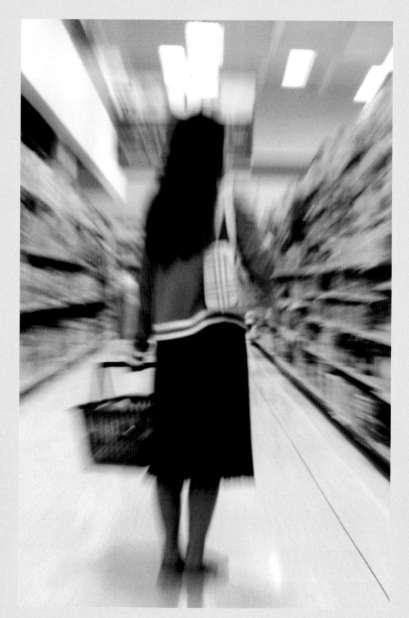

A person with kleptomania often does not know she's going to steal ahead of time. The impulse to take something in a store may come on her unexpectedly—and irresistibly.

People with kleptomania know that stealing is wrong and that their behavior would seem irrational or even absurd to others. Knowing that their behavior is wrong and illegal but feeling unable to control themselves leads many people with kleptomania to feel depressed, guilty, and fearful of being caught. Unlike people who steal because they want to or because they cannot afford something they need, people with kleptomania usually do not plan to steal ahead of time. Instead, they steal when the impulse urges them to do so, without prior thought to what they will steal or what the consequences will be. Although many people with kleptomania don't keep the stolen objects, some people will stash the objects away or try to secretly return them to the place from which they were stolen.

Although there is a lack of **conclusive** data on the subject, it appears that kleptomania can develop at any time between childhood and adulthood, but that it is rare for it to develop in late adulthood. Kleptomania appears to affect women more often than men.

There seem to be three ways in which kleptomania is experienced:

- **Sporadic.** A person with sporadic kleptomania has short periods of stealing separated by long periods of time in which she does not steal. The person, for example, may steal many things over the course of three days and then not steal anything for a year.

- **Episodic.** In episodic kleptomania, the periods of stealing are longer and separated by periods of not stealing. A person with episodic kleptomania may regularly steal objects for three months and then stop stealing for five months.

- **Chronic.** A person with chronic kleptomania steals on a regular basis. There may be periods of time when she steals more and periods of time when she steals less, but the stealing remains a habitual part of her life.

Pathological Gambling

Pathological gambling is a disorder in which a person gambles to such an excessive and uncontrolled extent that it disrupts his social, familial, and working relationships and functioning. Many people gamble, and many of these people may even gamble to excess but not have a pathological gambling disorder. According to the DSM-IV, to be diagnosed with pathological gambling disorder, a person must have five or more of the following characteristics:

1. The person is often absorbed in thinking about gambling, devising ways to get money to gamble with, strategizing for his next gambling venture, or reliving former gambling episodes.

2. The person needs to risk more money each time he gambles in order to feel the same excitement that he previously felt with less money.

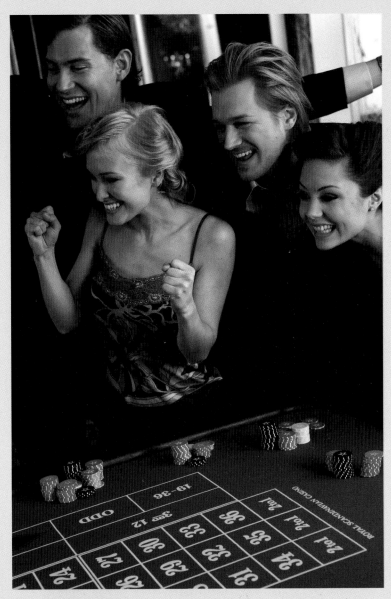

Many people gamble for recreation, and some people even do it as their profession—but the life of a person with pathological gambling disorder is completely overpowered with gambling to the point that it may destroy him financially and socially.

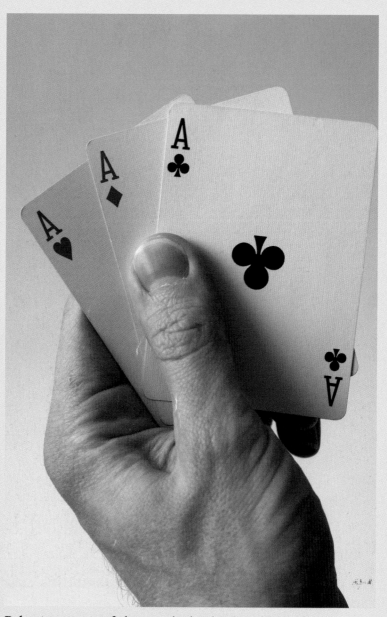

Poker is a growing fad among high school students. However, many adults are concerned about this trend. Research has shown that individuals who begin gambling as adolescents are more apt to have pathological gambling disorders as adults.

3. The person has tried on a number of occasions to stop or reduce his gambling but fails.

4. Attempting to cut back has a negative affect on the person's mood making him tense, peevish, or unpredictable.

5. The person uses gambling to escape from other stressful circumstances or emotional problems in his life. For example, the person might gamble to escape from thinking about problems at work, difficulties with his family, or to alleviate depression.

6. The person participates in a behavior known as "chasing one's losses" in which the person, after losing money gambling one day, returns the next day or soon after to try to win back the money.

7. The person lies about his gambling to try to keep others from knowing the extent of his behavior. Not only does the person lie to family and friends about his gambling, he might even lie to mental health professionals at the very same time that he is seeking treatment for his gambling.

8. The person has engaged in criminal activity, like theft or fraud, to get money with which to gamble.

9. The person's excessive gambling has caused him to risk or lose jobs, relationships, or other important positive aspects of his life.

10. The person's excessive gambling has led to debt or financial instability so serious that he needs to turn to other people for money or support.

Once it has been determined that a person's gambling behaviors meet five or more of these criteria, a doctor must also determine that the person's gambling is not part of a **manic** episode. People experiencing mania may engage in **binge** behaviors like excessive eating, drinking, gambling, exorbitant spending, extreme amounts of exercise, or other types of unrestrained activity. If someone's impulsive gambling is part of a manic episode, then the person does not have pathological gambling disorder.

Trichotillomania

Trichotillomania, also called TTM or trich for short, is an impulse-control disorder in which a person habitually pulls out her own hair, causing significant hair loss. As with other impulse-control disorders, a sense of tension or internal disruption precedes the impulse to pull hair, and this tension is relieved once the impulse to pull the hair has been satisfied.

When considering a diagnosis of trichotillomania, a doctor must determine that the individual's hair loss is not caused by another medical condition like a serious rash, infection of the skin and hair follicles, or genetic hair loss. Many children go through short phases of behaviors like nail-biting and hair-pulling, so a doctor must also determine that the hair-pulling

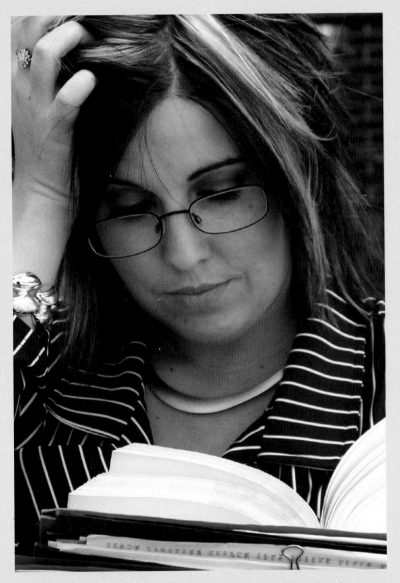

A person with trichotillomania may absently pull out her hair as she reads or watches television, releasing tension by engaging in this behavior. Since it can cause patches of baldness, this disorder can be particularly embarrassing for a young woman.

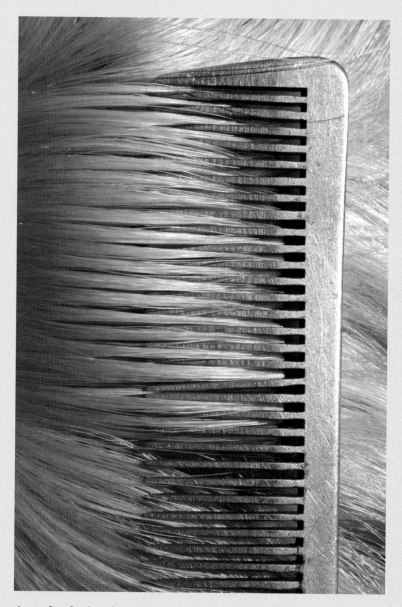

An individual with trichotillomania may be obsessed with hair—
to the point that she will examine hair, steal hair from other
people, and even eat hair.

is more than a short-term habit and is having a significant impact on other aspects of the person's life. For example, the individual's hair-pulling may have caused hair loss that is so noticeable that she is embarrassed to go to school, or long-term problems with hair-pulling and hair loss may lead to low self-esteem that keeps the person from participating in social activities.

Individuals with trichotillomania may be preoccupied with hair beyond pulling it out. They may closely inspect the pulled hairs, eat the hairs (a behavior known as trichophagia), or even try to secretly pull hair from other people. People with trichotillomania commonly have other habits, like nail-biting and skin-picking, and other disorders, like obsessive-compulsive disorder and eating disorders. If the hair-pulling is a direct result of another disorder, like obsessive-compulsive disorder, then the person should not be diagnosed with trichotillomania.

A person with trichotillomania might pull hair from any part of her body, but the most common places from which people pull hair are the head, eyebrows, and eyelashes. A common myth is that hair that is pulled out will not grow back. In very extreme cases of trichotillomania where the condition has existed for a long period of time, long-term damage may be done to the hair follicles, root, and blood supply. In most cases, however, a person's hair *will* grow back in its entirety once she seeks treatment and stops pulling.

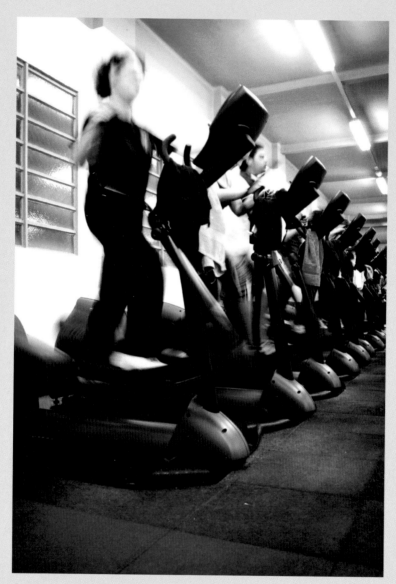

A person with an impulse-control disorder not otherwise specified might carry an ordinarily normal and healthy activity to extremes; for instance, she might become obsessed with exercising, to the point that exercise takes over her life, interfering with her social, emotional, and even professional life.

Impulse-Control Disorder Not Otherwise Specified

Explosive anger, stealing, fire-setting, gambling, and hair-pulling are certainly not the only ways in which people experience impulse-control disorders. The category impulse-control disorder not otherwise specified is given to patients who repeatedly fail to resist an impulse that is not one of the five impulses discussed above. Just as in the other forms of impulse-control disorders, the person's behavior must not be caused by another disorder (like obsessive-compulsive disorder or schizophrenia) and must be severe enough that it significantly impairs the person's regular personal, emotional, social, or occupational functioning.

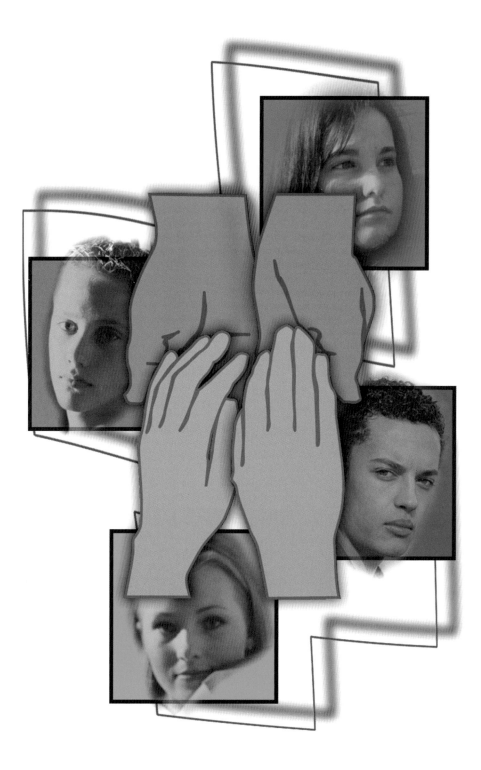

Chapter 3

The Little Turquoise Jacket

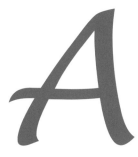n uneventful week has passed since Vanna's unnerving encounter with Ashley Gordon; little does she realize it is only the calm before a bigger storm. This Saturday afternoon Vanna is by herself, shopping at Westside Store Parade Mall.

Sometimes it feels good to get out of the South Shore neighborhoods and go where no one knows me she thinks as she sucks a frappuccino out of a straw and gazes at outfits in the window of Amandy's.

A little turquoise jacket catches her eye; she chucks the frozen coffee drink into a round trash receptacle and heads into the store's junior department. As she tries the jacket on, she thinks, *Sweet—it fits like it's already tailored for me!*

47

But almost immediately, she has that shaky feeling. *How can I get this jacket out the door?* She's wearing a tight little top with spaghetti straps; no way to put the jacket underneath that! She looks at her purse, a new little leather thing she lifted on Thursday; can't fit a jacket in that.

Sweating, her heart pounding, she heads toward the door. Dizzy, she puts a hand on a coat rack to steady herself; the room seems like it is spinning. She holds the jacket casually against her. *How am I going to get this jacket out of here?*

And then inspiration hits: *I'll just wear it out!*

Vanna walks through the lingerie department, pretending to look at panties while she makes sure no one is watching. *All clear—time to leave.* She strolls out of the store into the mall.

"Stop right there, young lady!" Seemingly from nowhere, a smartly dressed black man and a snippy-looking woman come alongside her.

They're store security officers! I can see the little microphones in their ears. I don't believe this.

"Put your hands behind your back please, ma'am." The male officer slips a set of plastic cuffs around Vanna's wrists.

Vanna feels like fainting or throwing up, maybe both. Her legs are so shaky she can barely stand, and she sinks to her knees, right there in the middle of the Pavilion with a crowd of shoppers staring.

What if someone from Shore View is here? There's bound to be someone in this crowd, or someone who knows someone. What will they say at school? I'll kill myself before I have to listen to their gossip. . . .

"Stand up please, ma'am" the female officer says, and somewhere Vanna finds strength to comply. They walk with her back through Amandy's and into a little office where a heavyset man is seated behind a big desk. The female officer pulls up a chair for Vanna to sit in.

"Nice taste," the man behind the desk says. "That little jacket has a $199.00 price tag on the sleeve. Too much for you to pay?"

Vanna stares at the floor while tears swell in her eyes. She shakes her head.

"Then why did you steal it?"

Vanna's voice is so faint she can barely hear her own words. "I don't know why."

"How many times have you stolen things?"

Vanna is still able to lie when she sees a strategic moment. "This is the first time, sir." She starts sobbing. "I don't know what came over me."

The man is silent for a few moments until Vanna regains her composure.

"Who are your parents?"

"Khan Rangsey and Khan Veata."

"Think they're home now?"

"Yes, sir."

"Call them and tell them what happened. Tell them to get over here right away." He hands Vanna a phone. She swallows back the bitter fluid in her mouth and punches in the number with her shaky fingers.

"Mae, I am so sorry. . . ." Vanna is crying too hard now to talk to her mother. But the man behind the desk is waiting. "I . . . I stole a jacket from a store. I am so sorry." Her voice cracks. "Please, Mae, the store security man wants you to come here. I'm at Amandy's, in the Westside Parade Mall."

Vanna hands back the phone and whispers, "They're coming. It will be a while—we live in Huntington Beach." Her shoulders slump.

After what seems an eternity, the Khans walk into the little office; their eyes are downcast. Vanna cringes as she sees the lines of shame that crease their faces.

"Mr. and Mrs. Khan, I am Joe Tanaka" the heavyset man says.

"Khan Rangsey," says Vanna's father and "Khan Veata," says Vanna's mother. The men shake hands; Vanna's mother keeps her hands at her side in the traditional Cambodian way.

"We caught your daughter stealing this jacket. It costs almost two hundred dollars."

Vanna's father shakes his head. "I do not understand. We give her many fine things."

"She said she could afford it." Mr. Tanaka looks at Vanna. "She may have a mental problem."

Vanna's mother says softly in a broken voice, "But sir, we are an honorable family."

"Yes, Mrs. Khan, you look like fine people. But some of the very best families—even Hollywood celebrities—have this sort of problem. I've seen it before in my line of work. Mr. Khan, your daughter says this is her first time shoplifting. Do you believe that is true?"

"Oh, yes."

"Then we don't need to trouble the police about this incident. You three may go now—but we don't ever want to catch your daughter shoplifting again."

An hour later, Vanna is seated in her living room in a black leather chair, facing both her parents on the sofa. She imagines herself in a cage suspended over boiling lava, and then thinks, *No, that's nothing compared to this torture.*

It isn't the fear of punishment that torments Vanna. Her mind conjures up scenes from the past that she has not seen but has heard described many times: her parents as a young married couple, running to escape from the napalm fire consuming their village . . . hiding and eating grubs in the jungle . . . crowded in a boat, praying for mercy from pirates that could rape or kill them. Vanna can never forget the perilous path her parents took to begin a new life in America, and she knows her mother suffered especially during these ordeals because she carried a little baby girl inside her through it all, a baby that would be Vanna.

"Vanna, what were you thinking?" her father asks.

Her head is bowed as she replies. "I was not thinking. Father. I am so sorry."

"What about your little sister?" asks Vanna's mother. "M'liss has many temptations at school now. What will happen if she sees her big sister is a thief?"

"I am so, so sorry, Mae. I didn't think about M'liss."

Her father speaks again. "I wonder Vanna, could this be our fault? Perhaps we have made mistakes raising you in this country. In the old land it was easier. Everyone shared the same ways in our old village. People knew the *dhamma*, the way of the Buddha and of truth. They followed right understanding, right thought, right speech, and—this is where you have failed today, Vanna—right actions."

He pauses, giving Vanna space to reflect, and then says, "Could it be that we lost our values living in all this plenty? We gave you expensive things—television, clothes, a car—

because we saw our neighbors do these things for their children, and we wanted you to be happy. But we have not done so well teaching you about spirituality and right behavior—and these are the most important aspects of life."

Again he pauses, so Vanna has time to digest his words. "Vanna, do you feel something lacking in your soul? Is that why you do this?"

Vanna doesn't know how to reply.

Then her mother asks, "Vanna, what are you going to do so this will not happen again?"

That's really the question, isn't it? Vanna thinks. *Heaven knows I don't want to do it again. If anyone saw today's incident my life is ruined. If I've been caught once I can get caught again. But how am I going to stop shoplifting?*

As soon as Vanna asks herself the question, she remembers her conversation with Ashley Gordon. For a long moment, she remains silent, thinking, and then she says slowly, "Mom, Dad, I think there may be a way for me to get the help I need. It's not the method of your—I mean our traditions, but maybe it can help me to find the path." She pauses to take a deep breath. "A girl at school told me about a doctor, a psychiatrist. She says Dr. Graham helped her with . . . emotional problems. I think that's what this is, an emotional problem, because it's really bad." She pauses, not sure how to continue. *Should I let them know the whole truth?*

Vanna sucks in a deep breath. "This isn't the first time I've stolen things. I lied to the man at the store. I've shoplifted many times. I really don't know how to stop myself or why I do it. There's something wrong inside of me." She raises her eyes and looks into her parents' faces. "Please, let me see this doctor."

Her parents are quiet for a long moment. Vanna's gaze sinks back to the floor in front of her, but finally, she can bear the silence no longer. When she looks back up into her parents' faces, she sees that their cheeks are streaked with tears.

Vanna's father says quietly, "Let us call Dr. Graham."

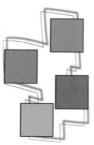

What Causes Impulse-Control Disorders?

Different areas of the brain are responsible for processing different types of information. For example, one part of the brain is responsible for long-term

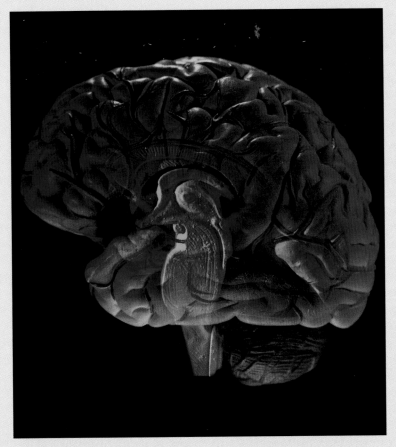

For your brain to do its job, all its parts must be communicating with each other. The brains of people with impulse-control disorders may not be able to carry out this communication normally.

memory. Another part of the brain is responsible for short-term memory. When you are learning a new lesson, a certain area of your brain becomes active. When you are engaged in physical activity, a different part of your brain is working. In order for you to function properly, all these different parts of your brain must communicate and share information with each other.

If you learned a new lesson today about the proper way to behave on a date and wanted to use that information to figure out what went wrong on your failed date last week, you would need the learning part of your brain to communicate with the memory part of your brain. Or imagine that your younger sibling does something to make you really angry, like ruins your favorite piece of clothing or rips every page out of your favorite book. The parts of your brain responsible for reactions and reflexes may surge to strike out at your sibling. The parts of your brain, however, that are responsible for learning lessons and maintaining beliefs and values access your belief that hurting others is wrong. The different parts of your brain communicate all these messages to each other, and you decided to take a deep breath and control your urge to hurt your sibling.

People with impulse-control disorders may have a lack of communication between these different areas of the brain. Messages between different parts of the brain are sent using chemicals called neurotransmitters. If the brain is not communicating properly, it could be the result of an imbalance of neurotransmitters or a malfunction in the parts of the

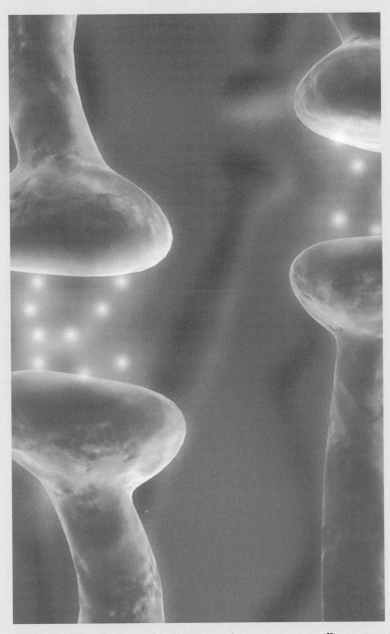

Neurotransmitters carry the messages between nerve cells.

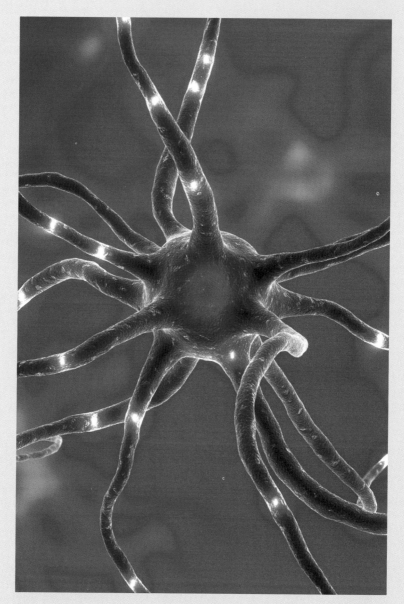

When nerve cells do not communicate normally with each other, various psychiatric disorders may be the result, including impulse-control disorders .

nerve cells that pick up neurotransmitters. Serotonin is one of these chemicals that play an important part in the communication between different regions of the brain. How well different regions of the brain are able to communicate with each other seems to influence the way we behave.

People with a high tendency toward aggressive and hostile behavior appear to have highly active sympathetic nervous systems and underactive parasympathetic nervous systems. Serotonin seems to play a large role in how these different parts of the nervous system function and communicate.

The sympathetic nervous system is responsible for the "flight-or-fight" response within the body—the immediate impulses you feel when faced with a stressful or dangerous situation. The parasympathetic nervous system balances, slows, and blocks the effects of the sympathetic nervous system in the body. For example, if you felt threatened by a person at school, your sympathetic nervous system would flood your body with hormones in preparation for a fight or a quick retreat. However, you know that it is better to solve problems calmly and rationally, so your parasympathetic nervous system would begin sending other messages to block the fight or flight response and calm your system.

One theory about the role of these systems in impulse-control disorders is that the sense of tension patients describe feeling prior to committing an impulsive act could be the result of an overactive sympathetic nervous system. The sense of relief they feel after committing the impulsive act may be

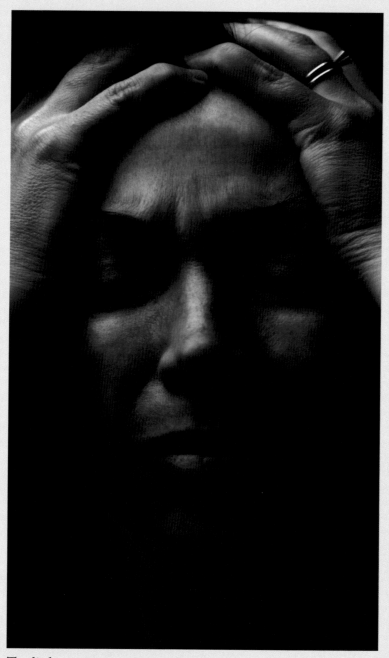

Too little serotonin can cause many problems, including depression and other mood disorders.

caused by the impulsive action "kick-starting" the parasympathetic nervous response.

Serotonin plays an important part in relaying the messages of the parasympathetic nervous system to the sympathetic nervous system. A person with too little serotonin tends to have an overactive sympathetic nervous system and underactive parasympathetic system, leading to a greater tendency toward impulsive behavior. Too little serotonin can also affect our moods, sleep, eating habits, learning, and many other important functions.

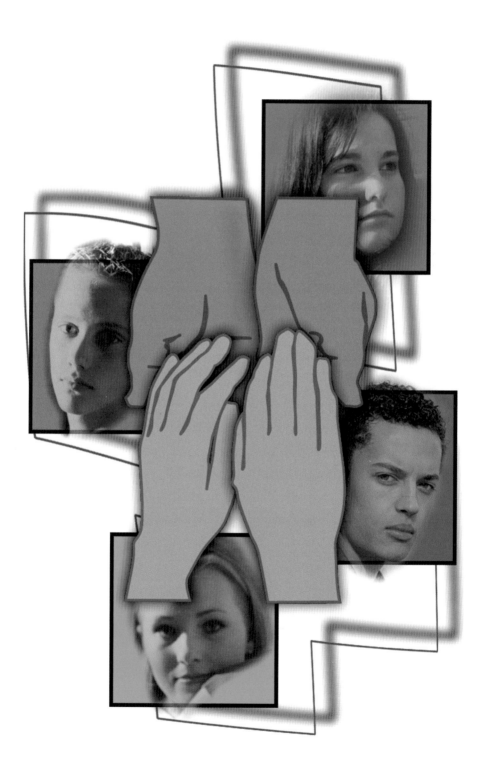

Chapter 4

Illumination

anna never thought she would actually visit a psychiatrist, and now that she is, it feels surreal. She stands in the hallway, staring at a door labeled *Dr. Monica Graham: Psychiatrist*. Finally, Vanna takes a deep breath and gives the door a shove. She steps into a small office and walks over to the receptionist window.

"Vanna Khan, here to see Dr. Graham." She speaks in a low voice, glancing around to make sure the room is empty of other clients.

"Good morning, Miss Khan. Please fill out this form," the receptionist tells her.

Vanna fills out the paperwork and hands it back in, then glances through an *Elle* magazine while waiting. *What will*

*Dr. Graham be like? Probably some pushy, overbearing Cau-
casian woman, a real feminist-Nazi type. She'll ask all kinds
of embarrassing questions and then tell me my parents potty
trained me all wrong.*

The receptionist says, "Miss Khan, Dr. Graham will see
you now."

*I could just run out of this office and tell my parents I saw
the doctor,* Vanna thinks, but she forces her reluctant legs to
stand and propel her through the door.

The moment she enters, Vanna finds herself facing a
well-dressed, surprisingly young blond woman with a wide
smile.

"You must be Khan Vanna."

She understands Cambodian name etiquette—that's nice.

Vanna forces a smile and extends a hand, but her eyes
are downcast. "Pleased to meet you, Dr. Graham."

The doctor motions her to sit in an armchair and says,
"Oh, those are really neat earrings. Where did you find
those?"

Vanna feels immediately more comfortable. "There's
this weird little boutique in Laguna, on the corner of
Ocean and Palm." *No need to mention that I didn't exactly
pay for them.*

"Is that the place between Starbucks and Crystal Fanta-
sies?" Dr. Graham asks.

"Yeah." *This doctor is all right.*

"They have some pretty neat things, I like to shop there for variety," the psychiatrist says. Then she gets down to business, "Vanna, this chart says you have never visited a psychologist or psychiatrist before. Is that right?"

Vanna nods.

"You may be struggling some with the idea of talking to a mental health professional."

Vanna looks to the floor and nods more vigorously.

"Did you know at least half of all American families have a member who has seen a psychologist or psychiatrist? And my clients include all kinds of people."

"Any Cambodians?"

"Yes. And blacks, Latinos, Iranians, Armenians. Vanna, do you think that colds or the flu discriminate based on the status or race of the people they infect?"

"No."

"Mental health issues are just like physical health—they strike indiscriminately."

"Yes," Vanna says. "But what I do is . . . not like a cold. It's . . ." She stares at the floor and lets the word hang in the air.

"Embarrassing?" asks Dr. Graham.

Vanna nods.

"Vanna, what things are you afraid of?"

Vanna struggles to find an answer. "When I was a little girl," she says finally, "I didn't have much of a social life. My parents hadn't been in this country long. We spoke Khmer in the house, so my English was poor. When I went to school and the other children saw my clothes, heard my accent—they called me 'Gook' and 'Boat Girl.'" Vanna's eyes are starting to water, and the words are tumbling out of her mouth now, surprising her. "They laughed at me. It hurt so bad. I swore I'd show them. I'd dress right and talk right and no one would dare laugh at me."

"How has that worked out? Are you popular?"

Vanna smiles. "I'm in with the in crowd."

"I'm not surprised."

"That's why I'm so afraid. If someone learns about . . . ."

"About your kleptomania?"

"Yes, about the shoplifting. It's so trampy."

"It is trampy, but you still do it."

"Yes."

"Why?"

Vanna shrugs. "I have no idea. Really. I get all sweaty until I do it, and then I feel better afterward. It doesn't make any sense."

"Not to your rational mind," Dr. Graham says. "Have you ever heard of serotonin?"

"The stuff in my brain?"

"Yes."

"We learned about that in chemistry class. I got an 'A.'" Vanna is proud of her good grade. She knows some of the kids think she is an airhead—but she proved them wrong.

"Well, good. That'll help us to talk about this in an intelligent manner."

Dr. Graham goes on to explain impulse-control disorders and the physical causes of kleptomania—the uncontrolled impulse to steal. When the doctor finishes, Vanna lets out a long sigh. "So I'm not just . . . bad?"

"Vanna, you know shoplifting is wrong, and that's why you feel guilty—but there's a disconnect in your mind between thinking and doing. Your moral values can't control your actions. We can work with that, and I can help you find ways to overcome your disorder. It may not be easy. Talk therapy can be scary. You might have to deal with things that you'd be embarrassed to tell your parents or friends. Do you think you can do that?"

Vanna feels fear crawling down her spine, spreading through her limbs. She wants to run out the door. Instead, she shifts nervously in the chair. "I don't know but . . . I'll try. Anything is better than someone at school finding out I have this problem."

Dr. Graham nods as though she understands exactly what Vanna means. "We'll help you identify the kinds of situations that trigger the urge to steal something—and then we'll be talking about new ways for you to think and act when those situations arise. I'll teach you how to re-train your thought habits so that your actions will change as well."

"How?"

"It will take time. But you can learn to replace thoughts of stealing with other thoughts. Our actions spring from our thoughts, you know." Dr. Graham picks up a pen from her desk and turns it between her fingers. "And Vanna, there's something else. Your behavior has a physical cause—and there's a prescription medication that may be able to help you."

"What do you mean? There's a pill I can take that will make me stop wanting to shoplift?"

Dr. Graham shakes her head. "It's not quite that simple. There is no prescription treatment specifically for klepto-mania, but medicines developed for depression and other disorders sometimes help with this problem as well. Would you be willing to try a prescription to see if it lessens your desire to steal things?"

Vanna asks, "Does anyone have to know?"

"Just your parents. You can keep it confidential."

"Okay."

Dr. Graham reaches for a prescription pad, then looks up and smiles. "So, Vanna, was this hour as bad as you were afraid it might be?"

The girl sinks back in her chair and smiles a little. "No. I was pretty scared but . . . you're cool."

"Thank you, Vanna. You're pretty neat yourself. Same time next week?"

"I'll be here."

On her way to the parking lot Vanna thinks, *I wish I'd known all that stuff about kleptomania and my brain and how to get help a long time ago. It's like my life is finally starting to make sense.*

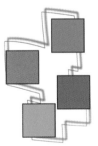

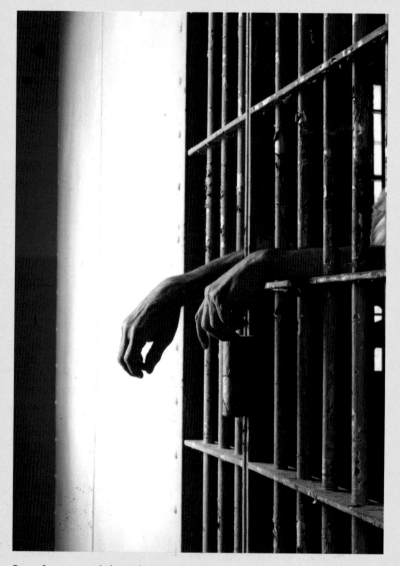

Impulse-control disorders can be at the root of some criminal behaviors; on the other hand, should an impulse-control disorder be reason to excuse a person from serving prison time? Sorting through these questions can be a difficult issue for the legal system.

Treating Impulse-Control Disorders

In the past, there was no treatment for people with impulse-control disorders because such people were assumed to be "common" criminals. In our society, people who harm others, steal, or set fires are usually put in jail or receive other legally determined punishments. Today, it is still all too common that people with impulse-control disorders are turned over to the criminal justice system instead of receiving medical treatment.

The problem of separating people with mental disorders from criminals is magnified by the fact that criminals sometimes claim to have impulse-control disorders in the hope of lessening their punishments or getting away with their crimes. For example, an abusive parent might claim to have intermittent explosive disorder to justify hurting his child, even though he does not have the disorder. When caught stealing, a robber might claim to have kleptomania, even though she does not. False claims like these lead to suspicion and doubt when people who really do have impulse-control disorders need help.

Many other cultural and social values encourage people to doubt the existence of conditions such as impulse-control disorders. For example, impulse-control disorders have many of the same characteristics as addictions. In most addictions, people are dependent on a substance. In impulse-control disorders, people are "addicted" to a behavior. The person "needs" to gamble, steal, or pull hair to function, the same way a smoker might "need" a cigarette to get through her day. Although many people are now realizing the benefits of medication in helping break substance addictions, for a long time people believed that the only way to overcome addiction was to quit "cold turkey."

Groups like Alcoholics Anonymous and others promote the idea that changing our behavior is a matter of willpower and depends on a person's ability to recognize her weaknesses and claim responsibility for her actions. Groups such as these have helped thousands of people and families through the struggles of addiction. They have also, however, played a large part in creating and promoting the idea that individuals can modify their behavior if they simply want to badly enough and that failure to modify behavior shows a weakness of character or desire. Beliefs such as these are, of course, not limited to the realm of substance abuse, but influence how people perceive and treat impulse-control disorders. Some people believe that just as a smoker should quit cold turkey, a person with an impulse-control disorder should also be able to quit her behavior cold turkey.

However, the more modern medicine learns about the human brain and body, the more we realize that nothing humans do is as simple as pure, conscious decision making. Every action you take is influenced by millions of internal and external factors. Even a seemingly mundane action like getting out of bed in the morning is the result of numerous social, environmental, physical, and psychological factors.

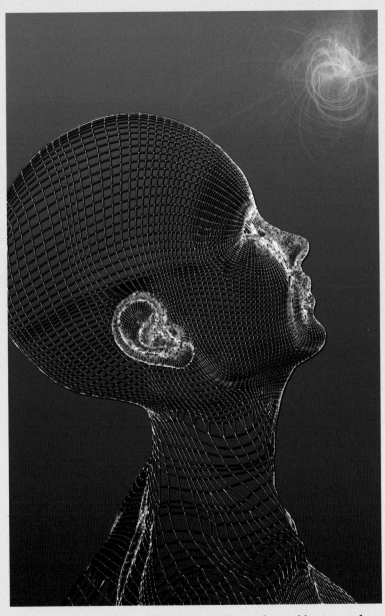

The connections between behavior and our physical brains and bodies are closer than people often suppose.

Your schedule for the day influences what time you decide to get up. The temperature, amount of sunlight, and weather conditions impact your body. The nutrients and substances from the things you eat and drink affect your *metabolism*. Things like stress and emotions affect hormone balances. Your body is absorbing and reacting to all these conditions and more, creating an infinitely complex mix of physical and mental factors that will ultimately determine

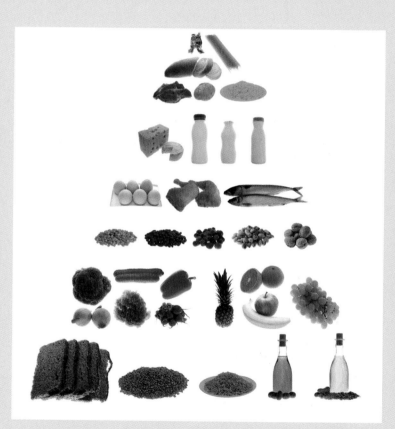

Eating a well-balanced and nutritious diet can help your emotional health as well as your physical well-being.

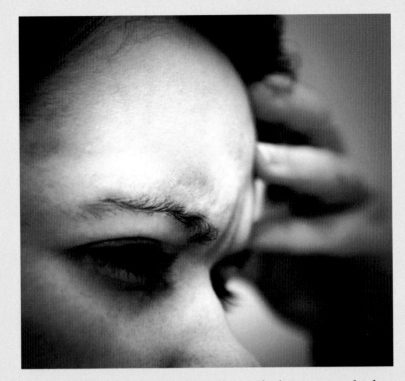

Stress can affect your hormonal balance, which in turn can lead to other psychological issues.

when you will wake and how you will feel when you get out of bed. Understanding that even simple daily decisions are part of a complicated web of physical and mental functions allows medical professionals to consider new perspectives and approaches when trying to understand more unusual behaviors like impulse-control disorders.

The main treatment method for impulse-control disorders has been psychotherapy, also called talk therapy. In individual therapy sessions, patients attempt to identify the emotional sources of their behaviors. The hope is that once the patient knows why he is behaving in a certain way, he will be able to change that behavior. Behavioral therapies show promise for treating impulse control disorders. Trichotillomania (the compulsion to pull out hair), for instance, can respond to behavioral therapies like habit reversal therapy or hypnosis. Pathological gambling may respond to twelve-step programs like Gamblers Anonymous, as well as cognitive-behavioral therapy and motivational enhancement therapy. In cognitive-behavioral therapy an individual learns to identify triggers for his or her behavior, to replace maladaptive thoughts and beliefs with more positive and proactive thoughts and to develop alternative behaviors. Motivational enhancement therapy offers an individual new reasons to behave in different ways.

The mind and body are connected in very intricate ways, however, and most peoples' actions cannot be traced to one factor. There are numerous mental and physical factors affecting everything we do, and the best treatments are those that can address all of the factors influencing a person's behavior. Although some impulse-control disorders might be treated most successfully through psychotherapy alone, growing evidence indicates there may also be chemical causes to these disorders. In such cases, medicines could be an important part of treatment.

One of the signs that impulse-control disorders may have significant chemical influences is that many people with impulse-control disorders suffer from **coexisting** disorders as well. For example, people

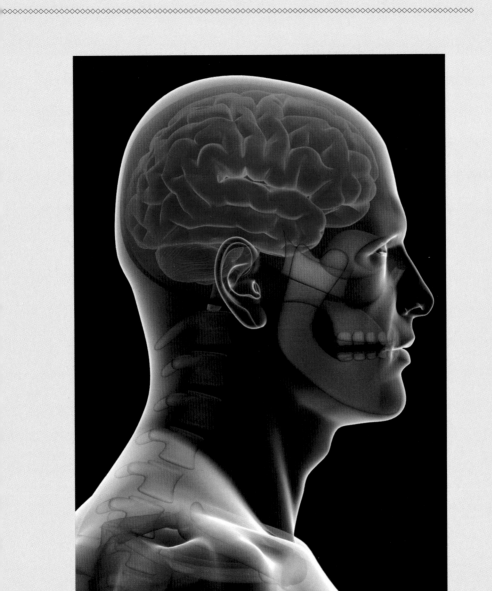

The mind and the body work together to shape who we are and what we do.

with intermittent explosive disorder sometimes describe physical sensations like tremors and head pressure before an explosive episode. They may have a history of migraine headaches, poor coordination, altered serotonin metabolism, and other disorders like mood disorders, eating disorders, and substance abuse. People with kleptomania and trichotillomania also have a high incidence of coexisting disorders, especially eating disorders (like **bulimia**) and obsessive-compulsive disorder. Many people with pyromania (the compulsion to light fires) are addicted to alcohol or have family histories of alcohol abuse, and people with pathological gambling often have histories of conditions such as hyperactive symptoms, mood disorders, and substance abuse. Recognizing these types of additional symptoms and conditions in people with impulse-control disorders has helped researchers identify possible drug treatments for these disorders. For example, some mood-stabilizing drugs, such as Depakote®, have been shown to help people with migraine headaches. In such a case, a medical researcher may see that some people with intermittent explosive disorder have a history of migraine headaches and mood disorders. The researcher may then think that, if this medication provides relief for mood disorders and migraine headaches, perhaps it will be helpful in treating intermittent explosive disorder as well. Depakote and other mood-stabilizing drugs have, in fact, helped some people with impulse-control disorders like intermittent explosive disorder and pathological gambling.

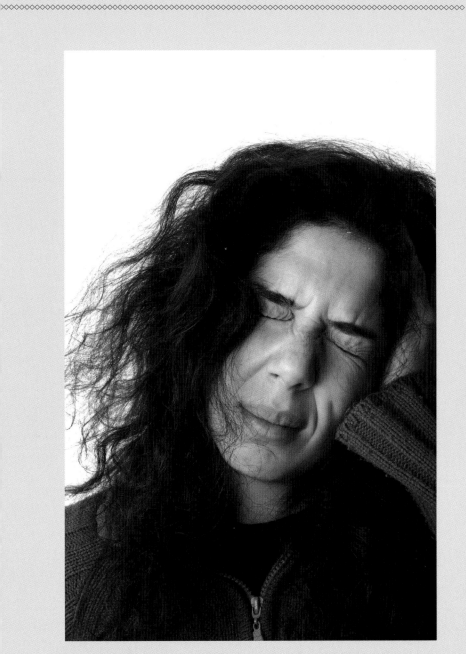

The same chemical and physiological issues that cause migraine headaches may also contribute to some impulse-control disorders.

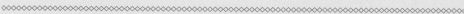

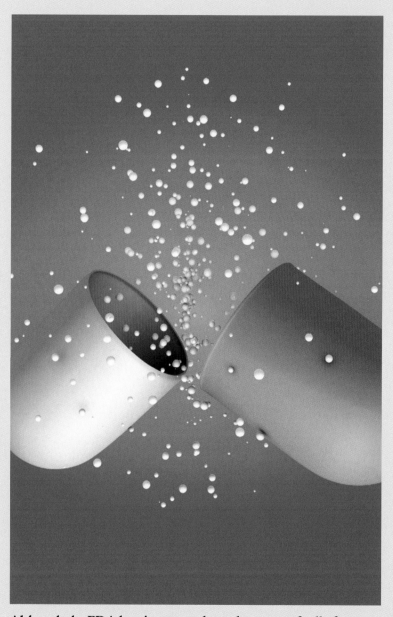

Although the FDA hasn't approved any drugs specifically for treating impulse-control disorders, some research seems to indicate that certain psychiatric medications may be helpful.

At this time, the United States Food and Drug Administration (FDA) has approved no drugs for the specific treatment of impulse-control disorders. However, many international studies and anecdotal evidence suggest that certain psychiatric medications help patients with impulse-control disorders, and research in this field is growing.

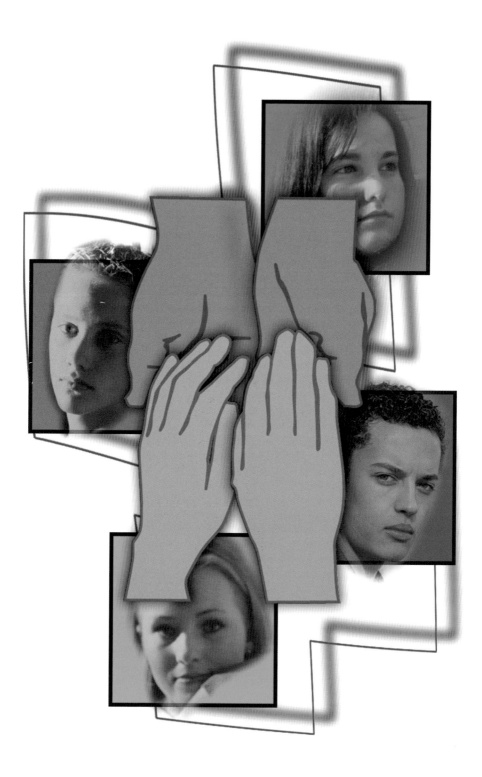

Chapter 5

The Truth About Kyle

Vanna has been feeling that her life is finally starting to make sense—but it's about to take a startling turn.

On Monday afternoon, she walks down the empty school hallway, having just left a meeting of the Shore View High Service Club. *It's a silly activity, but it will look good when I apply to UCLA. They care a lot about extracurricular activities. Service Club and candy striping at the hospital make me look like a real good citizen.*

As she strolls along the corridor, she pulls a set of tiny headphones from her purse, sticks them in her ears, and presses a button on her MP3 player. As she listens to a new song by Jason Hughes' band, she finds herself thinking about Jason.

He's awful shy for this screaming punk rock image he has. In fact, he's too shy to ask me out. But what would I say if he did? My life has too much drama already, without dating some-one people say is a heroin addict.

Her thoughts are interrupted as she walks past an empty classroom and something catches the corner of her eye. She stops to look through the window of the closed door. A figure is crouched in the corner of the room. *That's not the janitor. Who is it? What's that in his hand? It looks like a lighter. Oh my gosh.*

Vanna stands frozen in the hallway. *I could run to the office. But it might be nothing and I'd be totally embarrassed. If I confront this person, they could get violent. Then what? But I do have pepper spray in my purse. I'll go in there and see who it is, and keep my right hand on the spray in my purse, and I'll keep my distance.*

She takes a deep breath, turns the knob, and enters the room. The figure in the corner leaps to his feet and spins around to face her. *Kyle Brown! He's holding a cigarette lighter in one hand and a small can of lighter fluid in the other, and behind him there's this pile of papers and stuff.*

Vanna approaches Kyle warily, her right hand gripping the pepper spray in her purse.

"Uh, hi, Vanna," Kyle says, as though there's nothing weird about what he's doing. "What are you doing here?"

Vanna frowns. "Kyle, are you starting a fire?"

"What? You're crazy! What are you talking about?"

"You have a lighter and starter fluid in your hand. It's pretty obvious."

The two teens glare at each other for a tense moment; then suddenly, Kyle dashes for the door.

"No, you don't!" Vanna steps in his path, whips out the pepper spray, and aims at his face. "Another step and you'll feel such pain you won't be able to get out of the building. I'll scream, someone will come, and you'll go to jail."

Vanna's stomach is tied up in knots, but she plants her feet and squares her shoulders. She sees that Kyle is breathing fast, his eyes wide. They glare at each other for a moment that seems to last forever.

"Now what?" Kyle asks.

"You could tell me why you did it—last time, I mean—and why you're going to start another fire. Are you getting back at the school?"

Kyle gives a chuckle. "Nah. I've got nothing against school. Shore View High gives me something to do for eight hours a day. And besides, I learn lots of cool stuff in programming class."

"Then why—why start fires that cause damage and could hurt people?"

"I don't really think about that. It's just . . . well you wouldn't understand."

Vanna's nose wrinkles. "Try me."

"Okay," Kyle says slowly. "It just feels good. I'm thinking about fire all the time. I love to watch fires in my parents' backyard fire pit. I have favorite DVDs that I watch just for the fire scenes. It's an urge . . . I don't know. I think it's like wanting sex or something. Not that I'd really know. But I feel all tense and like I have to. . . . And then this—" He holds up the can of lighter fluid. "This is when I feel really alive. When I give in and start a fire. And afterward, I'm good for a few days. I feel okay for a while. But then, I need to do it again." Kyle pauses, his face red. "I guess that sounds pretty sick, huh?"

Vanna stares at Kyle with an odd mixture of fear and sympathy. "Kyle, I want to talk to you. I'm not gonna call anyone, at least not now. If I put the pepper spray down, do you promise not to run and not to hurt me?"

"I promise."

"For real?"

"I swear."

Vanna puts her arm down and relaxes her muscles, but she keeps the spray in her hand. "Actually, what you're describing isn't as weird as you might think."

"It's not?"

"Well, okay—most people would think it's weird, but I can sort of understand."

"Really?"

In her mind, Vanna hears her father's voice. *"The Buddha says, 'One should speak only to utter truth.' When you speak, Vanna, you should always speak out of the integrity within you."* Will Father's advice work here at Shore View High, facing an arsonist alone in a room? Maybe if I tell half a truth, that'll turn out best. Here goes. "Kyle, I have this friend who has a problem. She . . . shoplifts and doesn't know why. But she found this psychiatrist who understands and helps her. It seems like a moral problem, but she isn't really a bad person. It's a mental disconnect, something that has to do with chemicals in the brain. So . . . I can kinda understand your problem."

"Whoa! Vanna, the little rich girl, is a shoplifter?" Kyle looks both startled and amused.

"I didn't say me!" she screams.

"Yeah, yeah. Whatever."

Vanna frowns. "Look, Kyle. What you're doing is really dangerous. It costs other people a lot. I should turn you in right now, but I'm going to cut you a deal. I'll let you go, and I won't tell anyone what I saw this afternoon. But you have to do something, too. You have to get help. If you keep doing this, you're going to wind up in jail. Worse, someone could get hurt or killed because of your problem. So this is the deal, I let you go on condition that you promise me—promise me on whatever is most sacred to you—that you'll see a doctor or psychologist or someone to get help with this problem. And if there's another fire I swear your secret is out. You understand?"

He glares at her for a moment, but then he sighs. "Okay, deal."

"Swear to me."

"I swear to God—I swear on my mother's name—I won't start another fire and I'll go see a doctor about my problem."

"All right. Deal." Vanna backs out the door of the classroom, then hurries down the hall and out of the school. She feels like she has just woken from a nightmare. *Did all that really just happen in there? I'm shaking all over.*

She pauses in the parking lot, leans back against her Acura, and takes a deep breath. *I treated Kyle like I would want him to treat me if he saw me shoplifting. But this is serious. If he starts another fire, someone could get hurt. He better deal straight with me.*

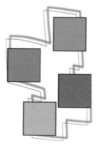

Pyromania

Pyromania is an impulse-control disorder in which a person purposefully sets fires. As in kleptomania, a person with pyromania feels a building sense of tension or unrest directly before setting a fire and feels relief or pleasure from setting the fire and observing the fire and its effects. Usually, the person is fascinated not only by fire but by other things

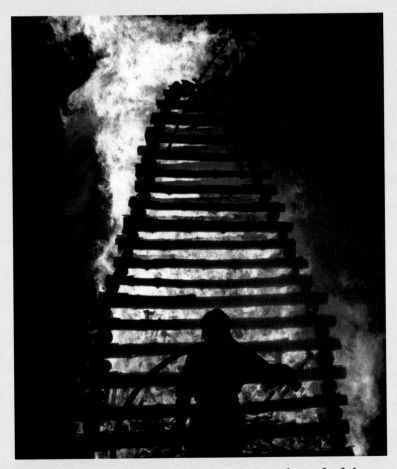

Occasionally, someone with pyromania may work as a firefighter to give himself more opportunities to be around fires.

having to do with fire, such as lighters, fire alarms, and fire departments. People with pyromania are so fascinated by fire and things associated with fire that they often even become firefighters so that they can be close to fire.

People with pyromania do not set fires out of anger, for financial reasons (such as being awarded insurance money for lost property), or to destroy evidence of other crimes. When considering a diagnosis of pyromania, a doctor must also be careful to determine that the fire-setting activities are not caused by other mental disorders (like **schizophrenia** or **conduct disorder**) and that the person was not acting with judgment impaired by **delusions**, hallucinations, alcohol, or substance abuse.

Unlike kleptomania in which people do not plan ahead to steal, people with pyromania often do plan to start a fire prior to carrying out the act. However, in this planning stage they may not consider the consequences, such as property destruction and harm to themselves or others. However, some people with pyromania feel **gratification** from the damage their fires cause.

Although fire-setting in children and adolescents is rather common, true pyromania is a rare disorder and occurs in males more often than in females. Most of the fire-setting done by young people is due not to an impulse-control disorder but to other external social influences or adjustment-related disorders. For example, young people may set fires because of peer pressure, as part of erratic behavior associated with attention-deficit/hyperactivity disorder, or because of

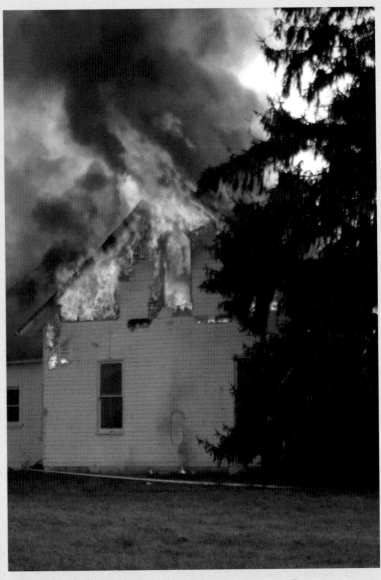

Neither the person who sets fire to his house to collect insurance from the loss nor the one who burns down her neighbor's house because she is angry has pyromania. A person with pyromania sets a fire simply because of the way it makes him feel.

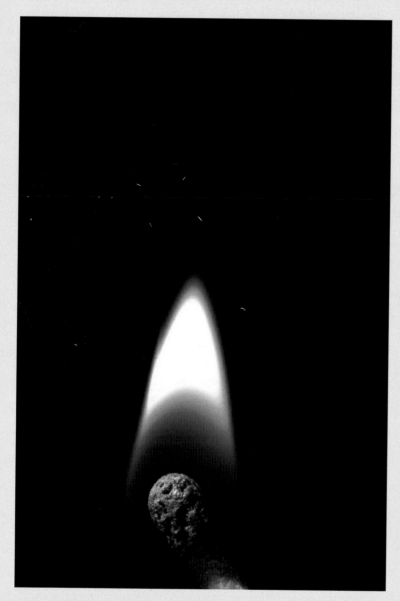

Almost all human beings, and particularly children, are fascinated to some extent with fire. A person with pyromania, however, is more than fascinated; he is obsessed, and setting fires gives him a sense of emotional release.

frustrating circumstances they do not know how to deal with **constructively**. It is also relatively common for young people to set fires simply by accident when experimenting with things like matches and lighters. An isolated incident of experimenting with fire or purposeful fire-setting is not a sign of pyromania.

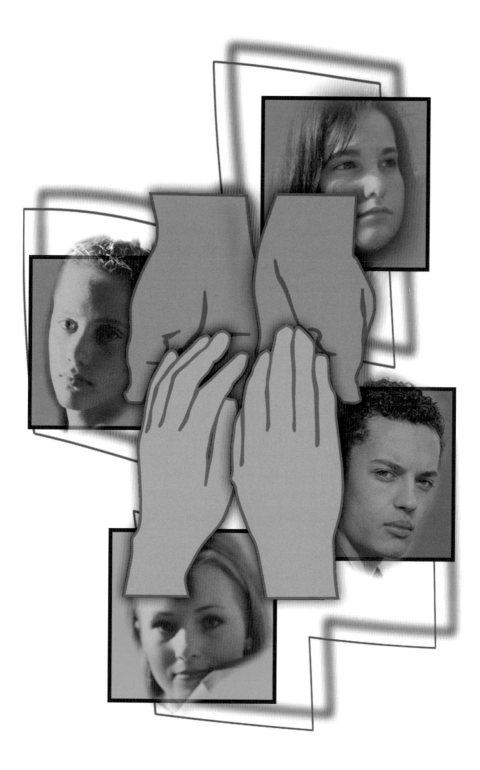

Chapter 6
Blackmail

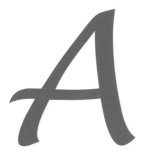week later, Vanna sits in English class listening to Mr. Sanchez teaching *The Scarlet Letter*. His style is "teaching through questioning," and discussion is an important part of students' grades.

"So class, what is Reverend Arthur Dimmesdale's big secret in this novel?"

Josh Bruner puts up a hand. "He was sleepin' with Hester Prynne and got her pregnant, but he won't tell because the Puritans think he's all righteous, and he won't ruin his reputation."

"Good answer, Josh. Hester Prynne can't hide her sin, since pregnancy is pretty obvious. So she has to wear a big scarlet letter on her dress every day. That's 'A' for adultery. What do you think of that form of punishment?"

Jaynee has a hand up. "It's so totally unfair. The woman gets blamed, and the guy gets away with it."

Jason Hughes has a hand up as well. The whole class knows that Mr. Sanchez dislikes Jason's comments; the lanky boy usually plays the role of class clown. Sanchez looks around, but no one else has a hand in the air.

"Yes, Jason?"

"I think Mr. Dimmesdale is a real dude."

"Thank you, as always, for your astute observations, Mr. Hughes."

Jason winks at Vanna, trying to impress her with his crazy attitude.

"All right," Mr. Sanchez says. "Let's look at this novel from another angle. Reverend Dimmesdale hides his sin, but Hester is forced to wear hers—which one is really worse off?"

Josh answers him. "Actually, in Hawthorne's view, the lying priest is worse off. The guilt of his unconfessed sin is killing him. Hester can deal with her past because it is out in the open."

"Excellent, Josh!" the teacher replies. "So that's a major point of the book—better to have your secrets known than try and hide them."

Vanna normally participates in English class discussions in order to keep her grade up, but today she is silent, lost in her own reflections. *What if they still punished people like the Puritans did? I'd have a big scarlet "S" for Shoplifter sewn on all my shirts. And Kyle, he'd have a big scarlet "A" just like Hester Prynne, only his would stand for Arsonist.*

So are we better off keeping our secrets hidden? If she wanted to, Ashley could ruin my reputation with a few words. But she doesn't and I'm grateful. And I could tell on Kyle and he'd probably go straight to jail, but he'd take my reputation down with him. They should write a novel about kids in our school. . . .

"Vanna, you're unusually quiet today. What do you think is the point of this novel?"

Vanna struggles to find something to say; she dares not voice any of her real thoughts. "Uh . . . Puritans were really bad in the fashion department?"

The class laughs, Mr. Sanchez rolls his eyes, and Vanna waits for him to say something sarcastic, but the teacher doesn't get a chance to speak.

RRRIIINNNGGGG. The clang of the fire alarm rips through the classroom. Students grab their books and bags and head for the exit.

Vanna's mind races. *Please, please don't let it be another fire. I don't want to have to deal with Kyle. I have enough trouble not walking out of stores with stuff and getting through my sessions with Dr. Graham.*

She walks beside Jaynee, joining the throng shoving through the main hallway toward the big front doors. She sees the principal and a teacher blocking the stairway at the end of the hall. Smoke pours up the stairs behind them. *Oh no!*

The wail of sirens shreds the air as students step blinking into the sunlight outside the school. To her dismay, Vanna sees not only fire trucks but an ambulance zooming ahead of the other vehicles. A pair of EMTs jump out as soon as it stops and run into the school. Vanna's hand covers her mouth. *If someone is hurt, it's my fault. I could have prevented this fire if I'd told on Kyle when I caught him.*

A security guard is nearby, talking into her cell phone. Vanna runs over. "Mrs. Pao, is someone hurt?"

"Well, I shouldn't be telling you this, but since you two are friends—" Vanna's heart skips a beat as Mrs. Pao continues. "It's Stacie Combs. She was trapped in a room for a few minutes after it caught fire and has some bad coughing from smoke inhalation. The nurse is with her and thinks she'll be all right, but of course we can't take any chances with a student's health."

Vanna feels her eyes fill with tears, and the world seems to spin. Mrs. Pao puts her hand on Vanna's shoulder. "Send some good thoughts toward your friend."

Vanna sits down on the grass and puts her head in her hands. *Stacie's hurt and it's my fault.*

As she looks up, she sees a familiar figure walking toward the parking lot. Suddenly energized by rage, Vanna leaps up and runs after him, then cuts in front of him and blocks his path. "Kyle! We had a deal."

"I couldn't help it, Vanna. I just had to do it."

"Did you ever see a psychologist?"

Kyle laughs. "How am I going to get my parents to pay for a shrink?"

"Do you think this is funny?" Vanna is screaming now. "Stacie is going to the hospital in that ambulance. You started a fire and you hurt my friend. You're going down, Kyle Brown. The deal is off."

Vanna turns back toward the school; it will only take a minute to grab a teacher or a police officer and tell them where the arsonist is.

"Go ahead, Vanna, make my day." Kyle flings his words at her. "It'll be worth getting arrested to see the look on people's faces when I tell everyone—and I mean everyone—that little miss goody-two-shoes Cambodian princess is a shoplifter. Are you ready to say good-bye to your reputation, Vanna Khan?"

Vanna stops in her tracks; she leans against a parked SUV to steady herself.

Kyle smirks at her. "I didn't think you could do it. You love your popularity too much. And I don't blame you. See ya 'round."

He walks calmly to his car, gets in, and drives away. Vanna feels as if a thousand-pound weight is atop her, crushing her into the hot tarmac of the parking lot.

"So, Dr. Graham, I don't know what to do. I feel awful about what happened to Stacie, and Kyle is a real threat to other people's safety. But I don't know if I can live with my reputation ruined."

Vanna knows Dr. Graham is the one person she can count on to keep her secrets.

The psychiatrist's response is soft but straightforward. "Vanna, are you sure you don't know what to do?"

Vanna finds herself remembering a silly little thing that happened that morning. M'liss was shouting, "There's a spider! A big yickey spider!" and Vanna had taken off her sandal, ready to smash the eight-legged creature.

"Wait a minute, girls" their father said, scooping the spider onto a piece of paper. He took the spider outside and a minute later, he returned.

"Oh, Father." M'liss rolled her eyes. "It was only a spider. I can't believe you saved its life." She giggled.

Her father looked at his daughters. "Spiders may not be your favorite creatures, but they also have reasons for existence. Everything that lives has value whether we see it or not. Remember, girls, all life is sacred. It is our job to protect life whenever we can."

Vanna sighs now. She knows what her father would say she should do. "I have to call the authorities. Someone else may get hurt."

Dr. Graham nods and smiles.

But something else is troubling Vanna. "Dr. Graham, I think Kyle has a problem like I do. He doesn't think about setting fires as hurting people. He can't control himself."

"That's probably true," Dr. Graham says. "But you aren't helping Kyle any by covering for him. If he has an impulse-control disorder, the proper authorities can decide and address that. In the meantime, once he is apprehended, everyone at your school will be safer."

"I know that, Dr. Graham." Vanna sighs again. "What this comes down to is—I'm afraid of what I might have to face as a result of this. What if it ruins my reputation?"

Dr. Graham's smile is sad. "Sometimes, Vanna, we do the right thing and it still hurts."

The next day between second and third periods, Vanna heads for the staircase where the people who matter hang out. Despite all the stress of the preceding days, she is dressed impeccably as always. *Just because life is crazy, I'm not going to start looking like a bum.*

She sees her two best friends talking to one another. "Hi. Jaynee! Hey, Stacie, great to see you back in school."

They both turn and look at her coldly.

Oh-oh.

There's ice in Jaynee's voice as she says, "Vanna, from what I just heard . . . I'm not sure I really know you."

Stacie nods. "I was in study hall last period when two police officers walked in and took Kyle Brown away. He was shouting, and like fifty kids heard him. He yelled, 'Vanna Khan is in on this, too—she knew all about me lighting fires. And she's a freakin' shoplifter, steals stuff all the time. She sees a shrink because she's such a crazy klepto.' He kept shouting stuff about you all the way out the door."

Vanna feels suddenly sick to her stomach. She barely hears as Stacie yell, "You knew about Kyle! You could have stopped him. I had to go to the hospital. My lungs were all messed up with smoke because my supposed friend is hiding secrets for a crazy geek pyro. I hate you, Vanna! Don't ever call me again."

Stacie turns and stalks away. Jaynee stares at Vanna with hard shiny eyes. "Vanna, I always thought you were a put-on. There's the real thing, and there's the dime-store imitation. Now it's pretty clear what you are. You're just Cambodian boat girl trash." Jaynee turns slowly, to emphasize her dismissal of Vanna, and walks away.

As Vanna stands alone at the staircase, she can hear whispers as students pass by. "Did you hear about Vanna Khan? She's a shoplifter! Can you believe it?"

For the first time in her life, Vanna decides she can't go to her classes. She walks back to the school parking lot, gets in her car, and heads down the road toward the Laguna Beach shopping district.

Mom and Dad talk about karma, how what we do returns to us. Well I don't know about that. Seems to me no good deed goes unpunished.

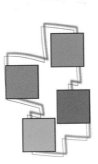

Impulse-Control Disorders and Medication

Some people have low serotonin levels because the cells that produce serotonin begin to reabsorb the serotonin before it can go out and perform its job in the body. This serotonin imbalance affects their moods and behaviors. Drugs called selective serotonin reuptake inhibitors (SSRIs) help to adjust this imbalance.

Though it is not clear exactly how SSRIs work, SSRIs like Prozac®, Paxil®, Zoloft®, Celexa®, and Luvox® appear to keep these cells from reabsorbing the serotonin. Preventing reabsorption allows the serotonin to stay in the body longer, hopefully leading to an increase in serotonin levels and an improvement in the patient's quality of life. SSRIs are prescribed to people with clinical depression because balancing serotonin levels helps to regulate a person's mood, but SSRIs have also helped people control eating disorders, alcoholism, smoking, aggressive behaviors, and obsessive-compulsive disorder (a disorder that shares many similarities with impulse-control disorders).

People with impulse-control disorders commonly develop clinical depression in addition to their other disorder; therefore, a doctor may wish to prescribe an antidepressant for this coexisting condition. Some antidepressants, however, can cause increased anxiety in the patient. Patients with impulse-control disorders mention tension and anxiety as factors that trigger their impulses, so doctors must be careful to

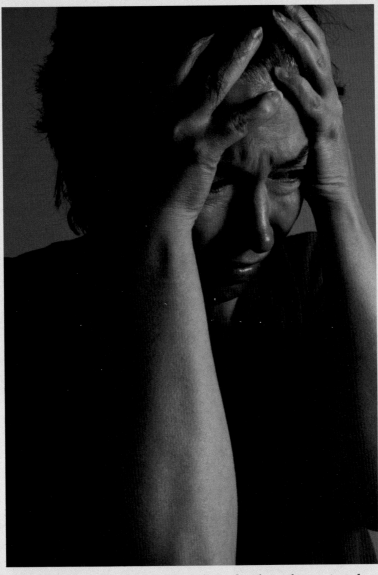

People with impulse-control disorders often have depression also. Taking an antidepressant to help them deal with their depression can give them the strength they need to address their impulse-control disorders as well.

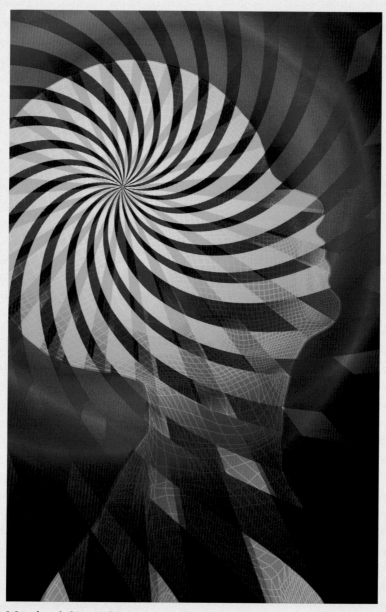

Mood stabilizers change brain chemistry, which in turn changes behavior. Scientists, however, do not understand exactly how or why these changes take place.

determine that a medication meant to be helpful will not end up making the patient's condition even worse. SSRIs tend to be a good choice should medication be needed because they have a low incidence of anxiety-producing side effects.

Although SSRIs seem to be the most promising drug treatment for impulse-control disorders, the class of psychiatric medications known as mood stabilizers has also helped some people with impulse-control disorders. Mood stabilizers are a group of drugs used to treat conditions such as mania and bipolar disorder. These drugs are also helpful in treating people with intermittent explosive disorder and pathological gambling disorder. Some of these drugs are also effective in the treatment of additional disorders like *epilepsy* and migraine headaches. It is not clear how most mood stabilizers, like lithium, and antipsychotics, like risperidone, produce their therapeutic effects. These drugs influence the chemical balance in the brain, but researchers do not yet know exactly how the drugs change chemical balances and why these changes affect behavior.

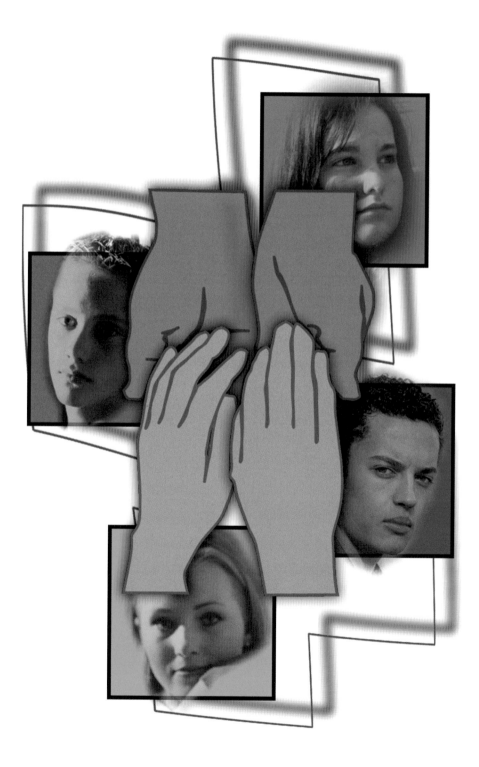

Chapter 7
Vanna's Choice

Vanna strolls slowly through her favorite shops, running her fingers over pricey jeans with hand-sewn sequins, blouses with fine stitching on the edges . . . the sorts of things that comfort her with their style and sheen.

Just past the public beach access, Vanna walks into Fashion Boutique. She looks at a table full of small accessories, and her eyes light on a wallet with a meticulously stitched image of Marilyn Monroe. *M'liss would just love that. She has this crazy thing for that old-time movie actress.*

Vanna's heart is pounding, her head spinning in the old familiar way. *No, that's my disorder I'm feeling. I don't have to pay attention. It's nothing worse than a headache really, just something quirky going on inside my skull. I'm taking the* medicines Dr. Graham prescribed; I've been working through my issues. That problem is better now.

But it's not. Vanna feels increasingly worse. After the horrors of rejection from everyone at Shore View High, she doesn't have the inner strength to say no to the craving that consumes her. *After everything that's happened to me in the last few days, I deserve a break. It's way too hard trying to be perfect.*

She glances around the store, scanning it out the corner of her eye. *No cameras visible, the woman that was behind the register stepped back in the room behind the store. Perfect.* One smooth move, and Vanna walks out of the store with the wallet in the bottom of her handbag.

She sucks in a long, slow breath and feels the tension ebb from her muscles. *Ahh . . . sweet relief.*

But her relief is short-lived. She hears her father's voice: *Perhaps we have made mistakes raising you in this country. In the old land it was easier. . . . People knew the* dhamma. . . . *They followed right understanding, right thought, right speech, and—this is where you failed today, Vanna—right actions.*

Vanna's purse seems to be getting heavier, as if the stolen wallet gains more weight every moment, dragging her down. She imagines giving the wallet to her sister, then remembers the words her mother spoke after the Amandy's incident: *What about your little sister? M'liss has many temptations at school now. What will happen if she sees her big sister is a thief?*

Vanna sits down on a bench and puts her head in her hands. *Too many people have been hurt because of my kleptomania. Mother and Father were ashamed to be dragged into a department store and told that their daughter is a thief. The man treated them nice, but I know it was one of the saddest moments of their lives. And there's Stacie. The smoke inhalation didn't do any permanent damage, but she must have been so scared, stuck in a burning room and her lungs filling with smoke. What more has to happen before I can control these impulses to steal things?*

Vanna closes her eyes, trying to practice mindfulness the way her parents taught her. She breathes deeply, stilling the voices in her mind, tuning out the world and all its craziness. She is still for several minutes. Then her own thoughts speak to her with a tone of quiet authority: *You are more than the clothes you wear, the car you drive, the things you own, Vanna. And you are more than your reputation. You have strength and intelligence you haven't even begun to tap into. You hold the power to choose.*

Vanna stands up and walks slowly back into the shop. "Ma'am," she says to the lady behind the counter, "I have a mental health issue—I'm a kleptomaniac. I just stole this purse from your store. I'm sorry. I'm returning it to you."

That night, Vanna accompanies her family to the temple where they worship. Her mother, father, and M'liss kneel beside Vanna before a large golden image of the Buddha, but Vanna has trouble keeping her mind on spiritual things. She recalls all the people who have cared for her, helped her through her problems.

Ashley Gordon could have told on me, but instead she referred me to Dr. Graham, and I still haven't thanked Ashley for that. Jason still has feelings for me, I'm sure. He has a problem; but so do I, and I'm improving, so maybe I can help him too. Dr. Graham has been a huge help; she gave me tools to handle this disorder before I got in worse trouble. And my parents have tried to show me the way to go, despite all the grief I've given them. Vanna's heart lightens. *My life is far from perfect—but it's looking brighter.*

She glances up from the floor toward the golden Buddha. He seems to be smiling at her.

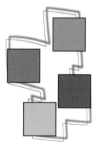

Alternatives and Supplements to Medication

Despite the fact that medications seem to hold hope for patients with impulse-control disorders, such medications are still supplements to the major treatment of psychotherapy. However, medication is not the only way that patients can supplement their therapy.

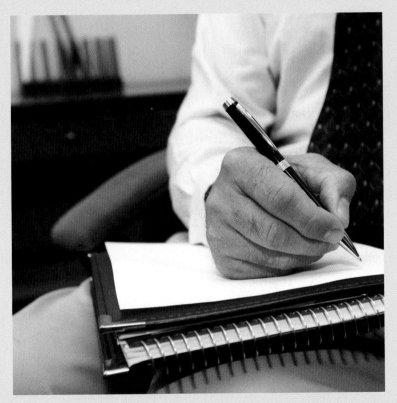

When you go for counseling, you will usually go through an intake interview where you are asked many questions about your physical and family background. This interview helps the counselor decide the best treatment plan to direct you toward.

One approach that can be helpful is group therapy. Though most therapists would not recommend group therapy as the primary source of treatment for a person with an impulse-control disorder, it can be very beneficial as an additional avenue of support. Many patients with impulse-control disorders feel alienated from other people. Their illnesses may cause them to feel isolated and to lose friends. In group therapy, patients can meet other people who are experiencing the same difficulties and who understand the hardships of struggling with an impulse-control disorder. Patients can find people who sympathize with their experiences. Because the people in group therapy are experiencing the same illness, patients can also be an important resource for each other, sharing information on doctors, treatments, lessons they have learned, and ideas for coping.

As with any treatment, group therapy also has its risks. Some group therapy sessions are run by trained professionals, while others are not. Some people may use group therapy as an outlet for frustration and negative feelings, turning what is meant to be positive into a negative experience. There is also the danger of becoming too reliant on the group therapy and losing the ability to cope outside the support network. As with all treatments, a patient should research carefully before entering into a treatment program.

Impulse-control disorders tend to have a great impact on patients' families and friends. For this reason, some patients might want to supplement their individual therapy with family therapy.

Few of us are all alone in the world, so when an individual has an impulse-control disorder it will affect his entire family. As a result, therapy may also help the whole family. It is easy to feel angry and resentful toward a person with an impulse-control disorder, but therapy can help family members understand the situation better.

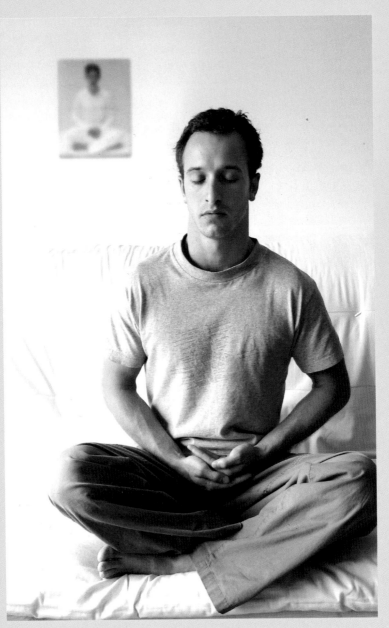

Yoga and other meditation practices may help a person with an impulse-control disorder handle stress in a more healthy way.

Many people find it helpful to supplement their major therapy with smaller therapeutic elements they can incorporate into their daily lives. For example, doing little things like stopping for a cup of tea during the day or relaxing in a hot bath with lavender-scented oil after work can do a lot to ease day-to-day stress and tension. Taking yoga and meditation classes can teach people valuable relaxation skills that can be called on in times of stress and crisis. For people with impulse-control disorders, a major goal of therapy might be to learn to handle the stresses of everyday life in order to reduce the likelihood of triggering impulsive actions.

In their book, *Anger Kills*, Redford and Virginia Williams give a list of seventeen "Survival Skills" for reducing hostile thoughts, feelings, and actions in your life. They are:

1. Reason with yourself.

2. Stop hostile thoughts, feelings, and urges.

3. Distract yourself.

4. Meditate.

5. Avoid overstimulation.

6. Assert yourself.

7. Care for a pet.

8. Listen.

9. Practice trusting others.

10. Take on community service.

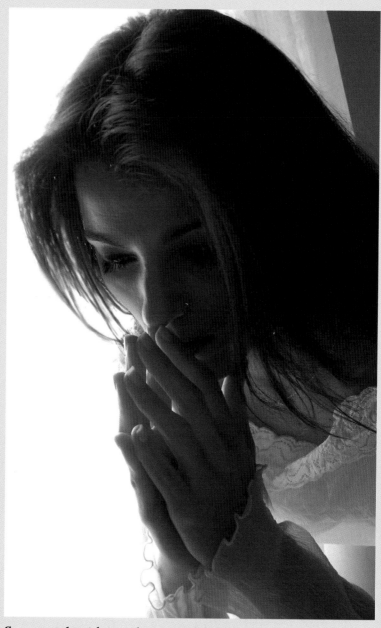

Some people with impulse-control disorders draw strength from faith and prayer.

11. Increase your empathy.

12. Be tolerant.

13. Forgive.

14. Have a confidant.

15. Laugh at yourself.

16. Become more religious.

17. Pretend today is your last.

Of course, the authors are giving suggestions to help people deal with hostile feelings, and these suggestions certainly are not cures for impulse-control disorders. In fact, some of these suggestions—such as reason with yourself and stop hostile thoughts, feelings, and urges—might seem almost impossible for a patient with an impulse-control disorder. However, making even a few of these adjustments can improve the quality of anybody's life. Even if not providing a cure, improving other aspects of one's life can make facing and dealing with impulse-control disorders easier.

Glossary

binge: Unrestrained or self-indulgent activity.

bipolar disorder: A psychological condition characterized by periods of extreme highs and extreme lows.

borderline personality disorder: A personality disorder characterized by difficulty in maintaining interpersonal relationships, instability of self-image, expressions of appropriate feelings, and control over impulses.

bulimia: An eating disorder characterized by periods of binge eating followed by periods of purging, such as self-induced vomiting and the use of laxatives.

chronic: Continuing for a long period of time.

coexisting: Being present at the same time as something else.

conclusive: Gives proof, resolves all doubts or disbelief.

conduct disorder: A behavioral disorder in childhood characterized by persistent violation of others' rights and age-appropriate social norms and values.

constructively: Describing an action that causes improvement or positive effects.

criteria: A test or requirements that must be met for making a decision.

delusions: An incorrect belief based on a misinterpretation of reality and that persists despite evidence that it is false.

epilepsy: A neurological disorder characterized by periodic physical or sensory seizures.

extenuating: Additional circumstances that may give partial justification for an act.

gratification: The state of feeling a sense of pleasure.

hallucinations: A sensory perception without evidence of its existence.

intermittent: Starting and stopping or alternating.

manic: Describes a state of abnormally intense activity that may be accompanied by extreme personality changes, violence, quickly alternating moods, or a dramatic sense of happiness.

metabolism: The chemical changes in the body that provide energy to the cells.

pathological: Something that is caused by a disease or repetitive, compulsive behavior that is so abnormally severe as to be characteristic of illness or disease.

Further Reading

Golomb, Ruth Goldfinger, and Sherrie Mansfield Vavrichek. *The Hair-Pulling Habit and You: How to Solve the Trichotillomania Puzzle*. Washington, D.C.: Writer's Cooperative of Greater Washington, 2000.

Haubrich-Casperson, Jane, and Doug Van Nispen. *Coping with Teen Gambling*, 1st edition. New York: Rosen, 2003.

Libal, Autumn. *Drug Therapy and Impulse Control Disorders*. Broomall, PA.: Mason Crest, 2004.

Wambaugh, Joseph. *Fire Love: A True Story*. New York: HarperCollins, 2002.

Williams, Julie. *Pyromania, Kleptomania, and Other Impulse Control Disorders*. Enslow: 2002.

For More Information

Gamblers Anonymous
www.gamblersanonymous.org

The Obsessive Compulsive Foundation, Inc.
www.ocfoundation.org

Psychology Information Online
www.psychologyinfo.com/problems/impulse_control.html

Shoplifters Alternative
www.shopliftersalternative.org

Trichotillomania Learning Center
www.trich.org

Publisher's note:
The Web sites listed on this page were active at the time of publication. The publisher is not responsible for Web sites that have changed their addresses or discontinued operation since the date of publication. The publisher will review and update the Web-site list upon each reprint.

Bibliography

Allen, Thomas E., Mayer C. Liebman, Lee Crandall Park, and William C. Wimmer. *A Primer on Mental Disorders: A Guide for Educators, Families, and Students.* Lanham, Md.: Scarecrow Press, 2001.

Cupchik, Will. *Why Honest People Shoplift or Commit Other Acts of Theft: Assessment and Treatment of "Atypical Theft Offenders."* Toronto, Ont.: University of Toronto Press, 2001.

Flannery, Raymond B. *Preventing Youth Violence: A Guide for Parents, Teachers, and Counselors.* New York: Continuum Publishing Group, 2002.

Healthinmind.com. "Pyromania (Compulsive Fire-Starting)." healthinmind.com/english/pyrom.htm.

Lepkifker, E., P.N. Dannan, R. Ziv, I. Iancu, N. Horesh, and M. Kotler. "The Treatment of Kleptomania with Serotonin Reuptake Inhibitors." www.biopsychiatry.com/klepto.htm

Psychological.com. "Impulse Control Disorders." www. psychological.com/impulse_control_disorders.htm.

Psychology Information Online. "Impulse Control Disorders." www.psychologyinfo.com/problems/impulse_control.html.

Psyweb. "Impulse-Control Disorders (N.E. Class)." psyweb. com/Mdisord/jsp/impud.jsp.

Index

Picture Credits

Authors

Kenneth McIntosh is the author of numerous books for teens. He lives in Arizona with his wife.

Phyllis Livingston has degrees in both psychology and special education. She has worked with many teens facing a variety of psychological disorders.

Series Consultants

Dr. Bridgemohan is an Assistant Professor in Pediatrics at Harvard Medical School and is a Board Certified Developmental-Behavioral Pediatrician on staff in the Developmental Medicine Center at Children's Hospital, Boston. She specializes in assessment and treatment of autism and developmental disorders in young children. Her clinical practice includes children and youth with autism, developmental language disorders, global delays, mental retardation, attentional and learning disorders, anxiety, and depression. Dr. Bridgemohan is Co-director of residency training in Child Development at Children's Hospital, Boston, and is co-editor of "Bright Futures Case Studies for Primary Care Clinicians: Child Development and Behavior," a curriculum used nationwide in Pediatric Residency training programs. Dr. Bridgemohan has also published research and review articles on resident education, toilet training, autism screening, and medical evaluation of children with developmental disorders.

Cindy Croft, M.A.Ed., is the Director of the Center for Inclusive Child Care (CICC) at Concordia University, St. Paul, MN. The CICC is a comprehensive resource network for promoting and supporting inclusive early childhood and school-age programs and providers with Project EXCEPTIONAL training and consultation, and other resources at www.inclusivechildcare. org. In addition to working with the CICC, Ms. Croft is on the faculty at Concordia University and Minneapolis Community and Technical College.